2nd Edition

Connecting with Grieving Clients

Supportive Communication for 14 Common Situations

LAUREL LAGONI, MS
DANA DURRANCE, MA

AAHA press

AAHA press

American Animal Hospital Association Press
12575 West Bayaud Avenue
Lakewood, Colorado 80228
800/252-2242 or 303/986-2800
press.aahanet.org

Library of Congress Cataloging-in-Publication Data

Lagoni, Laurel.
Connecting with grieving clients : supportive communication for 14 common situations / Laurel Lagoni, Dana Durrance. — 2nd ed.
p. ; cm.
Rev. ed. of: The practical guide to client grief : support techniques for 15 common situations / Laurel Lagoni. c1997.
Includes bibliographical references and index.
ISBN 978-1-58326-166-8 (pbk. : alk. paper)
I. Durrance, Dana. II. Lagoni, Laurel. Practical guide to client grief. III. American Animal Hospital Association. IV. Title.
[DNLM: 1. Bonding, Human-Pet. 2. Pets. 3. Communication. 4. Grief. 5. Professional-Patient Relations. 6. Veterinary Medicine. SF 411.47]

616.89'1658—dc23

2011034544

Book design by Erin Johnson Design

Printed in the United States of America

11 12 13 / 10 9 8 7 6 5 4 3 2 1

This book is dedicated to my wonderful family, who supports and encourages me even when times get tough. To my husband, Steve, your compassion and abilities as a practicing veterinarian are often the prototype of the very skills I'm trying to teach to others. Thank you for all that you do and for how much of yourself you give to your patients and clients. To Erin and Noah, thank you for inspiring me and always encouraging me to pursue my work even in the midst of chaos and craziness. You truly make my life shine. Finally, I dedicate this book to my sweet dog, Pfeiffer, who died this past year after 14 wonderful years in our family. We miss you, old lady, and love you very much. Keep rolling down the road!

—D. D.

I dedicate this second edition to YOU, the veterinary practice team. You make time every day to provide comfort and support for your grieving clients. You understand that tapping into the wisdom you possess is as necessary to the process of healing as using your medical knowledge and skills. Thank you for creating a "culture of caring" within your clinical environment and for paying special attention to your clients' emotional needs when their beloved pets die.

—L. L.

Contents

Acknowledgments

No book comes about in isolation. Two women, in particular, played important roles in bringing this one to fruition. I would like to thank Bess Maher, the American Animal Hospital Association's (AAHA's) acquisitions editor, for her guidance, enthusiasm, and friendship. Also deserving credit is Dana Durrance, my coauthor. Dana is always a willing writing partner and an endless source of knowledge regarding veterinary grief counseling. She makes writing seem easy! Thank you both for recognizing that this topic is vital to the success of every veterinary medical practice and for deeming this revision worthy of your time and effort. I also want to express my gratitude to the many veterinarians, animal health technicians, AAHA staff members, and reviewers as well as to many other colleagues who contributed to the revision and production phases of this project. Your insights and comments were invaluable, and the content and scope of this project are more realistic and usable because of them.

On a personal note, my gratitude extends to my coworkers at World by the Tail, Inc., who allowed me to write on "company time," and to my former coworkers at the Argus Institute for Families and Veterinary Medicine at Colorado State University's James L. Voss Veterinary Teaching Hospital. I learned all I ever needed to know about veterinary grief counseling with the tremendous support I was privileged to enjoy there. Thanks also to W. B. Saunders Company; Carolyn Butler, MS; and Suzanne Hetts, PhD, my coauthors on the textbook *The Human-Animal Bond and Grief*. Without their clinical innovations and collaboration over the past decades, many of the concepts in this book would not exist. —L.L.

For me, writing is often a roller-coaster ride replete with scary moments, unexpected twists, and tons of thrills. Ultimately, I always find the ride well worth the effort and can hardly wait to get back into the line again. First, I would like to thank my coauthor Laurel Lagoni for including me in this particular ride. I am never afraid of racing down that first steep hill when you're sitting beside me and holding my hand. Your understanding and patience got us through some of the more scary moments while making the thrills that much better. With each new writing project we share, I become more impressed with your insight, wisdom, and the camaraderie that we share.

I would also like to extend a huge thank-you to Bess Maher at AAHA for her unwavering support and for getting us on the roller coaster in the first place. Your talent and skills inspire me every day as well as your uncanny ability to translate what I'm thinking into the right words. It's a privilege to work with a person of such high character and I hope that we will continue to climb onto those roller coasters in coming years. Additionally, I would like to thank Iris Llewellyn for her guidance and expertise as well as the other editors and staff at AAHA for their expertise and hard work. I also extend my personal gratitude to all the wonderful and brave pet owners who have been willing to share their pain and grief with me over the years. You are the very heart and soul of the wonderful bonds we share with our companion animals. —D.D.

Preface

Everyone who loves a cat, dog, horse, bird, rabbit, or other animal deserves the opportunity to say goodbye in a meaningful and emotionally fulfilling way when the pet dies. You and each member of your veterinary practice team play a key role in ensuring that your clients are given these opportunities.

There are many ways that you and your team can truly *connect* with grieving clients and support them as they go through this challenging time. You can learn how to deliver bad news in a sensitive manner. You can learn how to teach clients about the many possible effects of grief. You can learn to conduct euthanasia in a way that helps clients who wish to be present when their pets die. You can learn how and when to use a variety of supportive communication techniques that will truly benefit your clients as they cope with loss.

In this book you will find descriptions of the clinical communication skills and supportive techniques that will best serve you and your clients in a variety of end-of-life situations. As a tool, it is designed for quick and easy access and is filled with suggested phrases and recommended actions that are clinically proven to work.

You can expect to achieve the following objectives by reading this book and practicing the skills it describes:

- Learn about the emotional effects of pet loss
- Increase your understanding of normal grief
- Add to your repertoire of client relations skills
- Increase your confidence about dealing with end-of-life topics
- Enhance your professional growth and feelings of personal satisfaction when your job requires you to "be there" for others

When connecting with grieving clients, there are few right or wrong answers or techniques; and a strategy that works well for one person may not work as well for another. However, there are supportive techniques that are *more effective than others* when dealing with typical pet loss situations and providing grief support. These are the strategies we've collected for you here.

How to Use This Book

> *Responding to grief in pet owners is an important measure of a veterinarian's humaneness."*
>
> —Steven Crow, DVM[1]

This book can be used as a personal preparatory or reference guide and as a training tool for practice team development.

A Preparatory and Reference Guide

The first time you read this book, be sure to read through all of the situations, paying close attention to the ones that are most similar to those you encounter in your veterinary practice. Don't stop with one reading, however. This book's usefulness only increases the more you review its contents and practice the techniques it describes.

When possible, use this book before meeting with clients who are in the midst of a situation involving grief, such as euthanasia of a pet. Review the situation presented in the book that best matches the client's situation. It will help you anticipate the emotional needs of your clients and prepare yourself to meet them, and you will feel more confident about providing them with comfort and support.

As you review the "14 Common Situations," you will see that the cases described are drawn from everyday scenarios found in general veterinary practice or emergency and specialty practices. Recording and occasionally reviewing the notes you take while reading will help you to develop your own unique vocabulary, client support style, and customized reference guide. Use the "Notes" section that completes each situation to write down the phrases, techniques, and protocols that work best for you and your clients. Then, you will have something to refer to when you are faced with similar situations in the future, and something to add to as you further develop your technique.

A Training Tool for Practice Team Development

Although the expression "experience is the best teacher" is true, it is not always a good idea to use real clients in real situations as a means of practicing and improving your grief support skills. Real-life experiences are necessary and inevitable; however, you can sharpen your skills before they arise by using this book as a source for developing role-plays for you and your team. Role-plays are a valuable way to train staff because they avoid the negative outcomes that can occur from practicing on real-life clients.

Role-Playing

Role-playing simply means acting out real-life situations with your colleagues during a practice session. Though it may sound simple and perhaps even artificial, role-playing can be the most effective way to teach, develop, and practice new, unfamiliar skills. Combined, the authors of this book have more than 40 years of experience training veterinary medical students and professionals to use grief support skills. In all that time, role-play has proven to be the single most important and effective teaching tool.

Role-plays usually involve two people, one playing the veterinary professional and the other playing the client. These two individuals then act out specific situations in front of others who become the audience and observe the action. There are many important reasons for and benefits to using role-play.

It's the next best thing to real life. You can read and talk about end-of-life protocols and client support methods for years, but until you actually *use and try on* these skills, they are never fully absorbed and solidified. Just as with surgery, or performing any medical procedure, you truly learn by actually *doing* the technique and then evaluating your experiences. If a picture is worth a thousand words, role-play "experience" is worth a million. When it comes to gaining confidence about providing grief support, there is simply no better method.

Little risk, big gain. Role-play provides a perfect way to teach and learn difficult material in a fairly safe, nonthreatening environment. If the person "playing" the role of veterinarian or veterinary professional struggles or makes mistakes, there's no real harm done, since real clients in real situations are not involved.

Creative learning means more successful learning. Role-play provides a unique and even fun way to learn new skills. It challenges you to go beyond your own perspective in a situation and see the other person's point of view. Role-playing often promotes group cohesiveness and positive energy. In fact, nationally recognized seminar trainer and management coach Micki Holliday believes that there are 10 reasons why experiential learning, such as role-playing, makes groups healthier and more positive:[2]

1. **Clarity:** Role-play provides and creates accurate communication scenarios by getting into detailed specifics.
2. **Supportiveness:** Role-play fosters a commitment among group members to encourage and support one another.
3. **Confidence Building:** Role-play encourages every member of the group to form a personal commitment to improving the self-image of *everyone else* in the group.
4. **Mutuality:** Successful role-play creates a partnership "orientation" where the outcome is win-win.
5. **Perspective:** Role-play allows employees to see things from differing viewpoints (from the perspective of the client, the employee, or even the boss), thereby increasing empathy.
6. **Risk:** Role-play encourages innovation and places emphasis on the effort made rather than the actual outcome. (Members are rewarded for taking a risk and being willing to try even if they are not successful.)
7. **Patience:** Role-play teaches patience, tolerance, and acceptance of individual communication styles.
8. **Investment:** The more involved group members become in a particular task, the more they will genuinely care about the outcome.
9. **Confidentiality:** Role-play teaches group members how to protect information exchanged in all team interactions and fosters a sense of trust and comfort with group members.

10. **Respect:** Role-play forces all group members to give and receive feedback, thus creating mutual respect all around.

When you begin to use role-playing as a training tool, it is important to set some clear and specific ground rules. Without rules and someone to enforce them, role-plays can accidentally take a negative turn and actually reduce trust among group members. Therefore, in the beginning it is best for the facilitator to be a hospital manager or supervisor. Once the group becomes comfortable, other staff members can act as facilitators. The following guidelines are essential for successful role-play and should be strictly enforced in a consistent manner.

Make it clear that everyone in the group participates. Whether one is playing the part as an "actor" in the role-play or is just an observer in the "audience," everyone has an important job. The actors practice new skills, while the audience watches and listens carefully in order to give constructive feedback.

Always ask for volunteers first. For all veterinary teams, the ultimate goal is for everyone to take turns at being actors and audience members. Explain that at first, many of them might feel nervous or shy when they are "on stage." Reassuring people that this shyness is common and goes away with time can reduce their discomfort. However, it is not a good idea to *force* a person to participate in role-play, especially if he or she is vehemently against it. Although these reluctant folks are often the ones who would benefit the most from the training, forcing the issue usually backfires. Instead, explain that each staff member who does not wish to role-play may simply say, "I pass," but after three passes, must find the courage to participate. If a particular person insists on passing more than three times, you may want to have a private conference to explore ways to encourage him or her.

Use "freezing" and "narrating" techniques. When the facilitator needs to interject something right away, she or he can simply say "freeze" to temporarily suspend what's going on in the role-play. The participants stop the action so that the facilitator may make an observation or ask a question. They can relax, however, while the comments are made; they do not need to remain in their poses. Freezing is also helpful if participants feel stuck, are struggling, or need help from the audience.

The facilitator might need to comment on the situation unfolding between the actors to keep the role-play on track. Through narration (which can be done during a freeze), the facilitator can share ideas with the audience about what the actors might be thinking or feeling in a specific situation. For example, "Client X is probably feeling overwhelmed right now after talking about euthanizing her dog. . . . What do you think would be helpful to do at this point?" Narration may need to be more leading for some situations than for others. If group members are to explore a new skill in a productive way, it is important for the facilitator not to narrate too much. If people are struggling or getting off track, do more narration.

Set specific guidelines and expectations. Tell the group that it is never okay to hurt anyone's feelings during role-plays even though some role-plays involve acting out conflict or an argument. Talk with group members about how they can determine if they are hurting someone's feelings (facial expressions, for example). Facilitate role-plays in a way that allows people the flexibility to truly try on new behaviors and issues that are important to them. This will create an atmosphere of trust, fun, and creativity. It is not helpful, however, to have role-plays that allow so much silliness that the message or the lesson is lost. The facilitator needs to be strong about keeping things on track (especially when the audience is giving feedback, a time when the conversation can digress to other topics).

One way to rein in the role-play is by making sure that people don't act out real-life, personal issues. Role-play is not the forum for such issues and is inappropriate (after all, this is not group or family therapy). Also, remind people not to overact or make the situation super-difficult for the actors. The idea is to try out new skills and help others learn them, not to put the actors through the ringer. It's okay if participants feel a bit of discomfort (that's how we all stretch ourselves and grow), but it's important not to take it too far. This is not theater; the idea is to mimic a real-life situation and practice communication skills.

Training by video is another way to learn new skills. There are two ways to use videos for this purpose. First, staff members can learn by viewing professionally produced videos designed to demonstrate effective techniques. Second, you can have someone videotape your own role-plays. When staff members view videotapes of themselves actually engaged in role-plays, they are able to *see* the effects of their words and nonverbal skills. They may notice facial expressions and body language they were not previously aware of. After viewing the tapes, it may be easier for them to understand the changes they could make in their interactions that might be beneficial to clients. When everyone on staff is videotaped and the tapes are viewed together, the role-play examples are more likely to be thought of as teaching tools. The contents become common ground for discussion.

Providing Feedback

Research indicates that new skills are best learned when instructors provide safe, supportive opportunities for practice.[3] In addition to the role-play itself, constructive feedback and debriefing sessions can help to accomplish this goal. Feedback is most beneficial when it contains the following elements:[4]

- **It is solicited rather than imposed.** Feedback is better absorbed when the receiver asks for the information rather than it being spontaneously provided by someone else.
- **It is descriptive rather than evaluative.** When the observer describes only his or her own reactions (descriptive), it prevents the person from feeling defensive and under attack. An example of descriptive feedback would be "I felt uncomfortable with the long silence between you. Was that uncomfortable for you as the client?" An example of evaluative feedback is "You let the silence between you go on way too long! Most clients would be uncomfortable in that situation!"
- **It is specific rather than general.** To tell an individual that he or she is dominating a situation is not nearly as useful as saying, for example, "When we were discussing things just now, I didn't feel like you were listening to what others were saying." Remember, if you have videotaped the role-plays, interactions like this can actually be *seen,* and therefore used effectively as teaching tools.
- **It is helpful to *both* the feedback receiver and the feedback provider.** Feedback can be destructive when it serves our own needs but fails to consider the needs of the person on the receiving end.
- **It is directed toward behavior that the receiver can change.** It is very frustrating when a person is reminded of shortcomings over which he or she has no control.
- **It is given in a timely manner.** Feedback is most useful when it is given shortly after the communication has occurred.

- **It is checked to ensure clear communication.** A way to check for clarity is to have the receivers try to rephrase the feedback they have just received to see if they have an accurate understanding of what was meant. If there is a misunderstanding, those who provided the feedback can clarify what they meant to say.

If you and your coworkers enjoy a fairly high level of trust and mutual respect, it might be interesting to use an actual case you're all familiar with as the basis of some role-plays. Role-plays like these often allow you to play yourself or a specific client (and gain some empathy for the client's point of view in the process). Participating in "real-life" role-plays can be intimidating, but sharing experiences, both rewarding ones and embarrassing ones, is a great way to learn from your own mistakes and successes as well as those of others. If you are secretive, defensive, and even modest about your own attempts to communicate with and help clients, little progress toward becoming more effective can be made.

Debriefing

During debriefing, it is important to ask questions that encourage the participants to think about and process what happened in the role-play. For example, "In this last scenario, what did the veterinarian do that indicated good listening?" "Did he [or she] do anything that indicated poor listening behavior?"

In general, a debriefing discussion should always begin with open-ended questions. The questions should become more specific as the participants' and observers' responses become more sophisticated. Let the group's responses drive the questioning. Good questions have the underlying message "I value your ideas and I want to know what you think." This helps maintain an atmosphere in which participants want to volunteer their thoughts, participate in discussions, and push themselves to use higher-order thinking and communication skills. Debriefing is more than venting your frustration. It means talking openly with your coworkers about your emotional experiences, as well as the medical aspects of a case, and then receiving constructive feedback and support regarding the communication techniques and course of action you chose to take. When you participate in a debriefing session, you can do the following:

- **Explain what you felt went well.** ("This technique really worked!")
- **Explain what you felt didn't go so well.** ("Mrs. James seemed to get angry with me when I suggested she might want to pay her bill ahead of time.")
- **Ask those present for ideas about other ways a situation might be handled.** ("How do the rest of you deal with suggestions that seem to offend clients?")

With time, even staff members who started out with trepidation about role-playing will find that the benefits far outweigh the drawbacks. As the shyness fades, confidence grows, not only in the role-playing itself but also in actual client situations. The new communication skills learned will become routine in day-to-day client interactions. Meanwhile, a greater sense of camaraderie among colleagues will develop. All of this will lead to a more fulfilling and rewarding daily experience for each member of the veterinary team. And, best of all, it will lead to better care for clients at the times when they most need understanding.

A Resource for Further Reading and Research

A list of helpful resources is included at the end of this book for readers who would like to know more about grief support as it pertains to veterinary medicine and companion-animal loss. In addition, there is a glossary for easy reference, providing ready access to definitions of the various techniques and skills in supportive language. Finally, Figure 1 is a sample role-play feedback form. This form is provided in the Appendix so you can make copies for yourself and team members.

Figure 1 Sample Role-Play Feedback Form

Name: Mary (veterinary technician)

Role-play situation: Helping Children (see Situation 10)

Mrs. Smith and her son, Jimmy, are having a tough time dealing with the death of their cat, Midas. Jimmy, in particular, is having trouble accepting it and is angry and upset. Mrs. Smith is also grieving but looking for support and assistance with how to help Jimmy. Mary is to offer her support to both Mrs. Smith and Jimmy.

Things that went well in the role-play:
(*to be filled out by colleagues observing the role-play*)

Mary, I think that you did a great job with a very difficult situation! You really jumped into the role-play and that's not always an easy thing to do. I really like how you acknowledged Mrs. Smith's and Jimmy's grief, avoided use of euphemisms, and weren't afraid to use the "death" word. I also think that you related to Jimmy on his level. Well done, Mary!

Ideas for improvement:
(*to be filled out by colleagues observing the role-play*)

It's difficult to tell parents how to talk to their children about death because you don't want to step on their toes, but it is appropriate to make suggestions and share your expertise. For example, you might have described to Mrs. Smith the things that you know are helpful for children and those that are, such as using euphemisms and not being truthful. Don't be afraid to give your direct opinion because often that is just what parents are looking for from you.

Thank you for being willing to participate in this role-play. Your effort has helped all of us to learn! Great work!

Signed,
Beth (client care specialist)

References

1. S. E. Crow, "Psychological Aspects of Veterinary Clinical Oncology," *Seminars in Veterinary Medicine and Surgery (Small Animal)* 1 (1986): 84–90.
2. M. Holliday, *Coaching, Mentoring, and Managing* (Franklin Lakes, NJ: Career Press, 2001).
3. P. K. Horvatich and K. B. Meyer, "Teaching Client Relations and Communication Skills: Part III—Preliminary Evaluations of Instructional Effectiveness," *Journal of Veterinary Medical Education* 7 (1980): 146–150.
4. S. M. Kurtz, J. Silverman, and J. Draper, *Teaching and Learning Communication Skills in Medicine* (Abingdon, Oxon, UK: Radcliffe Medical Press, 1998).

SECTION ONE

Connecting with Grieving Clients

Veterinary Grief Support

"Comfort, not health, is the primary and central objective of medical practice."
—Franklin McMillan, DVM[1]

Veterinary grief support has come a long way since the first publication of this book. When this specialized field emerged in the mid-1980s, grieving clients were often thought of as "overly sensitive," and providing pet loss support was considered extreme. Today, providing end-of-life care via Client Comfort Rooms, veterinary hospice programs, and client-present euthanasia is a standard part of daily practice.

The commitment to providing grief support for clients is due, in large part, to a growing recognition of the role the human-animal bond plays in people's lives. Surveys say Americans own 72 million dogs and 82 million cats, and almost half of all pet owners view their pets as members of their family.[2] Pets are often described as being like children or best friends, and the benefits they provide, such as emotional comfort, constant companionship, and unconditional love, are now widely recognized.[3]

The values and beliefs we hold about our pets have changed our relationships with them, and in turn, the pet-family bond has changed the daily practice of veterinary medicine. Today, pet owners know it is acceptable and healthy to express the love they feel for their pets and to grieve when their pets die; and they expect the members of their veterinary teams to help them through this grief.[4]

The death of a pet is often viewed as a significant and emotionally painful loss, with the grief and life disruptions experienced on par with the loss of a close friend or family member.[5] One study examined the grief responses of more than 200 middle-aged couples who had reported the death of a pet within the past three years. Of 48 life events, including the death of a spouse, divorce, marriage, loss of children, an arrest, loss of a job, and the death of a pet, researchers found, the death of a pet was the most frequently reported "trauma" experienced by the couples participating in the study. Survey participants said the death of a pet was less stressful than the death of a human member of their immediate family, but more stressful than the death of other human relatives. Forty percent of wives and 28 percent of husbands reported that the loss of a pet was "quite" or "extremely" disturbing.[6]

The impact of pet loss on human bereavement and the veterinary profession has been studied,[7] and popular literature also exists telling pet owners how they can deal with grief after their pets die.[8] However, there is relatively little information available for veterinary practice teams wishing to learn *how* to support grieving pet owners and help them cope with end-of-life issues such as decision-making surrounding euthanasia.[9] Since providing skilled, sensitive communication and support is almost a clinical requirement today, this is a significant gap—one that this book is intended to fill.

Loss and Grief

According to grief expert Murray Colin Parkes, "It is important for those who attempt to help the bereaved to know what is normal."[10] Developing an understanding of what normal grief looks like, as well as learning how to be comfortable with open (and sometimes dramatic) expressions of grief, helps you feel more confident about helping your clients manage their symptoms of grief. The textbox "Normal Expressions of Grief" provides an overview of the many ways normal grief can be expressed. A brief description of normal grief follows.

Normal Grief

As you begin to play a more active role in your clients' experiences with companion-animal death, you will find that most people know very little about coping with grief. You will also find that what they do know, or think they know, is generally inaccurate.

Research suggests that what people say and do during bereavement is often based on the myths and misinformation about grief that are passed

Normal Expressions of Grief

Although grief responses differ from one person to another, there are many predictable and normal ways for grief to be expressed. These expressions can occur on physical, mental, emotional, social, and spiritual levels all at the same time. Below are common symptoms of grief by category.

Physical
Crying, sobbing, wailing, shock and numbness, dry mouth, a lump in the throat, shortness of breath, stomachache or nausea, tightness in the chest, restlessness, fatigue, exhaustion, sleep disturbance, appetite disturbance, body aches, stiffness of joints or muscles, and dizziness or fainting.

Mental
Denial, sense of unreality, confusion, inability to concentrate, feeling preoccupied by the loss, experiencing hallucinations concerning the loss (visual, auditory, or olfactory), a need to reminisce about the loved one and to talk about the circumstances of the loss, a sense that time is passing very slowly, a desire to rationalize or intellectualize feelings about the loss, fleeting thoughts or fantasies about suicide (not accompanied by concrete plans or specific behaviors).

Emotional
Sadness, anger, depression, guilt, anxiety, relief, loneliness, irritability, a desire to blame others for the loss, resentment, embarrassment, self-doubt, lowered self-esteem, feelings of being overwhelmed or out of control, feelings of hopelessness and helplessness, feelings of victimization, shock, giddiness, affect that is inappropriate for the situation (nervous smiles and laughter).

Social
A desire to withdraw from others, a desperate desire never to be alone, feelings of isolation and alienation, a greater dependency on others, rejection of others, feeling rejected and misunderstood by others, a reluctance to ask others for help, change in friends or in living arrangements, a desire to relocate or move, a need to find distractions from the intensity of grief (to stay busy or to overcommit to activities as a means of escaping thoughts and feelings).

Spiritual
Bargaining with God in attempts to prevent loss, feeling angry with God when loss occurs, renewed or shaken religious beliefs, feelings of being either blessed or punished, searching for a meaningful interpretation of a loved one's death, paranormal visions or dreams concerning a dead loved one, questioning whether or not souls exist and wondering what happens to loved ones after death, the need to "finish business" with a purposeful ending or closure to the relationship (funeral, memorial service, last rites ceremony, or goodbye ritual).

along in families from generation to generation.[11] One of the most damaging of these myths is that the "right" way to handle loss is to be strong and stoic, never allowing grief to show. Another damaging myth is that staying busy and keeping one's mind off loss is the "right" way to quickly feel better and eventually recover. To avoid reinforcing these beliefs, it's important to become knowledgeable about the normal, healthy grieving process.

Loss and grief are two of our most common human experiences. However, until recently, conversations about loss, death, and grief have been taboo and viewed as morbid or morose. Thus, grief experiences haven't been openly discussed and shared, and we haven't built a common base of knowledge about the experience. Shared or not, the truth is that we actually know a great deal about loss and grief. Let's begin with some definitions.

Loss is defined as an ending or as a point of change or transition. Grief, or mourning, is the natural and spontaneous response to loss, the normal way to adjust to endings and changes.[12] It is a process, not an event, and is necessary for healing emotional wounds. It can take a long time to grieve a significant loss. There is no specific time frame in which the grieving process is completed. In fact, normal grief may last for days, weeks, months, or even years, depending on the circumstances of the loss. If this process progresses in a healthy manner, grief lessens in intensity over time.

Everyone has a unique response to loss, and there is no "right" or "wrong" way to grieve. Mourning can take different forms according to a person's age, gender, culture, and life experiences. For instance, women usually cry more often during grief than men.[13] Although tears are a complex mix of biological and cultural factors, men are socialized to maintain their composure during emotional times, while women are socially conditioned to express their feelings more openly.

Children can grieve just as deeply as adults, but, because of their shorter attention spans, they do so more sporadically.[14] Children most often express their grief through behaviors rather than through words. They act out their grief through artwork, play behaviors, or expressions of anger and irritability. Until they reach the age of eight or nine, children do not possess the cognitive development and language capabilities necessary to verbally express grief. However, their inability to verbalize grief should not be misconstrued for not feeling it. The loss of a pet is the first loss many children experience, and the confusion and emotional pain caused by it are very real.

Although grief is expressed in different ways, if it is progressing normally it does follow a fairly predictable course. There is an initial, acute phase of shock, despair, or denial; one or more middle phases of emotional pain and suffering; and a final phase of recovery.[15] As a veterinary professional, it is more useful for you to have a basic, working knowledge of the normal symptoms of grief than to have a great deal of theoretical knowledge about how grief progresses. This is because you are more likely to see your clients' grief when it is in the early, acute phases (e.g., during a medical emergency or immediately following a euthanasia) than you are to see it in the middle or final stages.

Anticipatory Grief

Your clients will be affected not only by the normal grief that follows loss but also by *anticipatory grief.*[16] Anticipatory grief occurs *prior* to an actual death and often begins with the diagnosis of a terminal illness or injury. As soon as a client senses that a beloved pet may die, he or she may begin to exhibit any or all of the manifestations of normal grief, as detailed in the textbox "Normal Expressions of Grief."

As the pet's condition deteriorates, the client must adjust to the changes. The pet's appearance, personality, and physical capabilities may change as a result of treatments or surgeries. The client may experience a sense of loss as it becomes necessary to give up knowing the pet in the old, familiar ways. During this period of anticipatory grief, clients begin the process of saying goodbye to their pets, with some consciously or subconsciously detaching from their pets (and perhaps moving quickly to euthanasia) and others clinging even more tightly to the relationship (and perhaps having difficulty making a decision about euthanasia).

Anticipatory grief is often characterized by anxiety, worry, guilt, confusion, and indecision. Sometimes clients who are in the midst of anticipatory grief are misunderstood and thought of as "difficult" or "problem" clients.[17] These are the clients who ask unending questions, doubt your competency, exhibit peculiar behaviors, or demand unreasonable access to you or to their hospitalized pets. "Problem clients" are often grieving clients, however, and their emotional states can usually be stabilized with an honest conversation about grief, along with your sincere emotional support and compassion.

Clients Who May Be At-Risk and Need Additional Support

Several variables can help you predict which clients may have more intense grief responses when their companion animals die. These clients may require more of your understanding and time and benefit from a referral to a mental health professional and/or a pet-loss counseling or support program.

- Cases that involve children. This includes teens and young adults who are away from home. The needs of older children are often overlooked when pets die.
- Clients who lose a childhood pet. This event often represents the "end of an era" for clients and can trigger other upsetting thoughts and feelings.
- Clients who live alone and cannot identify other sources of emotional support.
- Clients who say they "owe" their pet because the pet "got them through" a difficult period in their lives (divorce, domestic abuse, a previous loss). These clients may have a particularly difficult time with decisions about euthanasia.
- Clients who have recently experienced other significant losses and/or stressors (e.g., death of a family member, major illness, divorce, loss of a job).
- Clients who may be clinically depressed or those who make references to suicide, homicide, abuse, or other types of violence.

As a veterinary team member, you can best support your grieving clients by encouraging them to talk openly about their grief-related thoughts and feelings. You can also give a client "permission" or encourage him or her to grieve by letting the client know that you understand the need to cry, to ask questions, to be present at the pet's euthanasia, to view the pet's body after death, and to reminisce about the pet's life.

While it is unrealistic to expect you to provide long-term grief support for clients, high-quality veterinary care does include identifying clients who may be at higher risk than others for a more complicated grief response. See the textbox "Clients Who May Be At-Risk and Need Additional Support" for keys to identifying these clients. Although all grieving clients can benefit from information about pet loss and grieving, your "at-risk clients" are the ones who would most benefit from referrals to a credible, experienced grief support program or mental health professional in your community. Making informed referrals requires you to be familiar with your local community resources. A sample referral form for keeping track of these programs and professionals is included in the Appendix.

- Clients who identify their companion animal as being like a son or daughter or being their "only" friend or primary source of emotional support. Also, clients who anthropomorphize (assign human characteristics) to their pet to an extreme degree.
- Clients who "rescued" their pet from death or near-death (e.g., who prevented an accident that would have harmed the pet, provided previous treatment for an injury or illness in the pet, or adopted the pet from a shelter).
- Clients who have invested significant time, energy, and money in a pet's long-term medical treatment and now seem to have a difficult time "letting go."
- Clients who link their pet to another person, relationship, or time in their lives. These symbolic links often stem from previous losses that are unresolved and in need of healing (children who have died or moved away, significant relationships or marriages that have ended). Symbolic links also can stem from a meaningful time in a client's past (i.e., past experiences outdoors, such as hiking, fishing, and camping) or the client's hopes and expectations for a brighter, happier future (retirement in the mountains with plenty of leisure time together).

Supporting Your Clients' Grief

According to one study in human medicine, the leading reason for seeking medical care is *relief of distress*. The effort to minimize distress is often described in the medical literature as the act of providing comfort. Comfort means "to strengthen" and is most often described as a physical, mental, and/or emotional state of ease or well-being.[18]

In a 1998 commentary in the *Journal of the American Veterinary Medical Association*, Dr. Franklin McMillan suggested that comfort, not health, is the "primary and central objective of medical practice."[19] Dr. McMillan proposed that the purpose of fighting disease is to provide and maintain comfort, and that health professionals should view the elimination of disease as the single most important part of eliminating distress and discomfort.

If you think like Dr. McMillan, you know that, even when your patients die, you can still make a difference in your clients' experience by simply comforting them during those first painful moments following their loss. You provide emotional comfort when you listen to your clients' *nonmedical concerns* without taking action to solve their problems. This means acknowledging your clients' losses, creating opportunities for their thoughts and emotions to be openly expressed, and simply listening to their pain, as well as to their happier memories, if and when *they are ready* to share those with you.

Your clients possess the knowledge and skills they need to heal their own grief. When providing support for grieving clients, it's more helpful to simply empathize and listen than to offer advice about what you think your clients should do.

Listening is an overlooked support skill in veterinary medicine. As a professional, you might feel that you aren't being helpful unless you know the "right thing to say" to "solve" or "fix" your clients' dilemmas. Yet, the truth is, you can't "fix" grief. You can't cheer up your clients or make their feelings go away. Nor should you. Grievers need to *feel their feelings* in order to heal. Therefore, comfort is most helpful when it is offered as small gestures of support or by simply being a silent presence and witness to their sorrow.

Skilled emotional support is based on empathy and a genuine understanding of what your clients are going through. Empathy means having an intellectual and emotional comprehension of another person's condition without actually experiencing the other person's feelings.[20] The classic concept of "putting yourself in someone else's shoes" is an example of empathy. You convey empathy when you say, "I can imagine how sad you must feel, knowing that Samson might die."

Empathy is not sympathy. Sympathy is feeling sorry for someone. You are conveying sympathy when you say, "Poor Susan! I feel so bad for you." Expressing sympathy or pitying someone is not helpful when dealing with grief. Feeling pitied by others often offends people and can be counterproductive to feeling supported.

Setting Limits for Support

Veterinary team members who provide skilled client support often develop an extremely loving and loyal clientele. Many of your clients will think of you as a friend.

Once they have experienced the quality of your comfort and care, they may naturally turn to you for assistance with the other problems in their lives, especially when those problems involve a medical issue or death. For

What NOT to Say, What NOT to Do

Most of our knowledge about the "best" ways to deal with loss are based on myths and misguided information passed down from one generation to the next. And most of this information is just plain wrong! The following tips are based on years of clinical research and our experience with grievers and represent the interventions that have not been found to be helpful.

- Do ***not*** use clichés such as "time will heal" or "everything happens for a reason." Clichés are simplistic solutions to complex problems, and using them tends to make people suppress, rather than express, their feelings of grief.
- Do ***not*** compare one griever's loss to another's. Comparisons are attempts to minimize the impact of a loss and imply that the loss wasn't as bad as it could have been. Comparing one loss to another tends to make people suppress, rather than express, their feelings of grief.
- Do ***not*** encourage grievers to stay busy and to keep their minds off their grief. Grievers need slow, empty, alone time to fully experience their grief and move through it.
- Do ***not*** encourage grievers to make major changes in their lives. After a significant loss, many grievers consider moving, divorcing, or quitting their jobs. In general, though, grief clouds a person's judgment. Decisions made too soon after a loss may be regretted later.
- Do ***not*** attempt to cheer up grievers. Encouraging grievers to take vacations, go shopping, or medicate their pain with alcohol or tranquilizing drugs encourages them to avoid reality. Avoiding the immediate symptoms of grief can ultimately lead to complicated, unresolved, and even pathological grief outcomes.
- Do ***not*** scold or give advice, lectures, or pep talks to grievers who are feeling down. Grief is a process that can take weeks, months, and even years to complete. Grievers need patience and understanding from their friends and family members, no matter how long their feelings seem to linger.
- Do ***not*** suggest grievers replace the one they've lost. People who have experienced a loss are often urged to get on with life by remarrying, having another child, or adopting a new pet as soon as possible. Most grievers view this advice as insensitive and are deeply offended by the implication that anyone else could take the place of the unique and special loved one who died.

example, they may come to you with questions about an illness they are coping with, their child's struggle to recover from a severe injury, or the death of one of their close relatives or friends. These conversations will be emotional, and it will be tempting for you to try to help them as much as you can.

Basic Principles for Providing Effective Grief Support

It is not uncommon for caring, compassionate veterinary professionals to become overly involved in some of their cases. You must guard against this to avoid burning out. You will be of little help to your clients if you are so exhausted that you cannot focus on their needs. When you find yourself "in too deep," remember the following points about how you can provide effective help for others and still preserve your own sanity and sense of well-being.

- You cannot control how clients respond to loss or how they grieve; you can only control how you respond to your clients.
- Emotional support is useful only when it is accepted. If your assistance is clearly not wanted, back off.
- People have a right to feel whatever they feel, whether or not you think their feelings are right. Never try to take away someone's feelings or change one feeling into another in order to make your clients feel better. Simply acknowledge the feelings they describe.
- Always behave toward your clients with integrity and according to a code of ethics. In other words, respect your clients' right to confidentiality; convey information in honest, truthful ways; refuse to censor, lie, or withhold information in order to protect your clients' feelings; refrain from taking advantage of your clients' vulnerable emotional state; and always speak to clients with sensitivity and empathy.
- Know your personal and professional limits and never attempt to exceed the confines of your client-support role. Seek guidance or support from other professionals you trust when you need it.

If you begin to feel burdened by others' problems, gently remind yourself of the limits of your client support responsibilities. Remember that you are not a psychiatrist, psychologist, social worker, family therapist, member of the clergy, or suicide prevention counselor. Nor do you want to be! These are professional roles that require years of study and experience. You are, by choice, a veterinary medical professional and therefore required to deal only with the thoughts, feelings, behaviors, and issues associated with losing a beloved pet. While it is very appropriate for you to be sensitive and supportive, your efforts can be consistently limited to addressing the issues that arise surrounding the death of a companion animal.

If you have the time, it is always appropriate to listen to the problems of a "friend." But, if you find yourself drawn to help a "client-friend" attempt to resolve another personal issue, remind yourself that you may not be the best-qualified person to do so. This is the time simply to listen to your friend and then, if appropriate, make a referral to a mental health professional or local support program that can provide the specific kind of counseling your client-friend needs.

Please take care of yourself and remember that, when providing support, it is always more helpful to allow the other person to remain in control of his or her situation. Facilitate the grieving process by offering your clients guidance, structure, and honest information and by teaching them about what they can expect from the normal process of grieving. Emotional support efforts are most effective when you understand that you have a responsibility *to*, rather than *for*, your clients. It may be easier for you to understand the difference and to adhere to the limits and boundaries that define "support," as it relates to professional relationships, when you study the basic client-support principles, as well as what is *not* helpful to say or do, as described in the textboxes "Basic Principles for Providing Effective Grief Support" and "What NOT to Say, What NOT to Do."

References

1. F. D. McMillan, "Comfort as the Primary Goal in Veterinary Medical Practice," *Journal of the American Veterinary Medical Association* 212, no. 9 (1998): 1370–1374.
2. *U.S. Pet Ownership & Demographics Sourcebook* (Schaumberg, IL: American Veterinary Medical Association, 2007).
3. L. Lagoni, C. Butler, and S. Hetts, *The Human-Animal Bond and Grief* (Philadelphia: W. B. Saunders, 1994).
4. Ibid.
5. G. Gage and R. Holcomb, "Couples' Perceptions of the Stressfulness of the Death of the Family Pet," *Family Relations* 40 (1991): 103–106; B. H. Gosse and M. B. Barnes, "Human Grief Resulting from the Death of a Pet," *Anthrozoös* 7 (1994): 103–112; L. A. Planchon, D. I. Templer, S. Stokes, and J. Keller, "Death of a Companion Cat or Dog and Human Bereavement: Psychosocial Variables," *Society & Animals* 10 (2002): 93–105.
6. Gage and Holcomb, "Couples' Perceptions."
7. Ibid.; B. Fogle and D. Abrahamson, "Pet Loss: A Survey of the Attitudes and Feelings of Practicing Veterinarians," *Anthrozoös* 3 (1990): 143–150; L. A. Hart, B. L. Hart, and B. Mader, "Humane Euthanasia and Companion Animal Death: Caring for the Animal, the Client and the Veterinarian," *Journal of the American Veterinary Medical Association* 197 (1990): 1292–1299; Gosse and Barnes, "Human Grief Resulting from the Death of a Pet"; L. A. Planchon and D. I. Templer, "The Correlates of Grief after Death of Pet," *Anthrozoös*

9 (1996): 107–113; Planchon et al., "Death of a Companion Cat or Dog and Human Bereavement."

8. W. Sife, *The Loss of a Pet: A Guide to Coping with the Grieving Process When a Pet Dies* (New York: Howell Book House, 1998); B. J. Carmack, *Grieving the Death of a Pet* (Minneapolis: Augsburg Fortress, 2003); G. Kowalski, *Goodbye Friend: Healing Wisdom for Anyone Who Has Ever Lost a Pet* (Novato, CA: New World Library, 2006).
9. Lagoni et al., *The Human-Animal Bond and Grief*; S. F. Nakaya, *Kindred Spirit, Kindred Care: Making Health Decisions on Behalf of Our Animal Companions* (Novato, CA: New World Library, 2005); C. Barton Ross and J. Baron-Sorensen, *Pet Loss and Human Emotion: A Guide to Recovery* (New York: Routledge, 2007); M. D. Pilgrim, "Communicating Social Support to Grieving Clients: The Veterinarian's View," *Death Studies* 34 (2010): 699–714.
10. M. Parkes, *Bereavement: Studies of Grief in Adult Life* (New York: International University Press, 1972).
11. Owen Lipstein and Hara Estroff Marana, "Loss Loss Loss: An Interview with University of Chicago's Froma Walsh," *Psychology Today*, July 1, 1992, 64–94.
12. W. J. Worden, *Grief Counseling and Grief Therapy: A Handbook for the Mental Health Practitioner* (New York: Springer, 2008).
13. W. H. Frey and M. Lanseth, *Crying: The Mystery of Tears* (Minneapolis: Winston Press, 1985).
14. Lagoni et al., *The Human-Animal Bond and Grief.*
15. T. A. Rando, *Grief, Dying and Death: Clinical Interventions for Caregivers* (Champaign, IL: Research Press, 1984).
16. Worden, *Grief Counseling and Grief Therapy*; Rando, *Grief, Dying and Death.*
17. Lagoni et al., *The Human-Animal Bond and Grief.*
18. M. Brecht, "Nursing's Role in Assuring Access to Care," *Nursing Outlook* 38, no. 1 (1990): 6–7; J. Moseley, "Symposium on Compassionate Care and the Dying Experience: Alterations in Comfort," *Nursing Clinics of North America* 20 (1985): 427–438; W. W. Skeat, *An Etymological Dictionary of the English Language* (Oxford, UK: Clarendon Press, 1980).
19. McMillan, "Comfort as the Primary Goal in Veterinary Medical Practice."
20. *The Pocket Oxford Dictionary* (New York: Oxford University Press, 1992).

Clinical Communication Skills and Emotional Support Protocols

Most grief support is conveyed through the use of a specific set of basic clinical communication skills and techniques, including the spoken word and nonverbal behaviors like direct eye contact, touch, facial expressions, and body language. If you want to connect with and provide support for your grieving clients, it helps to be a skilled communicator. But skilled communication does not just happen; basic verbal and nonverbal skills and techniques can be learned, often through trial and error, but more effectively through education and practice. This section introduces some of the most important skills and techniques used in effective communication. Practicing these, and learning to apply them through the "14 Common Situations" presented later in this book, will allow you to reduce the "trial and error" part of the equation. With practice, every member of your veterinary team will become skilled in providing grief support.

When encountering situations involving grief, it also helps to have a plan. A grief support plan or protocol provides direction for your entire practice team. Written and well-rehearsed protocols help you and your staff understand *who* is responsible for each step of the client support process, as well as *when* each step should be implemented.

The outline shown in Figure 2 has been used in well-established clinical teaching programs and can be used to design client-support protocols for your practice. Before adapting your own protocols to this outline (also provided in the appendix "Forms"), it is useful to identify the purpose (e.g., client-present euthanasia) of the plan you are creating.

Figure 2 Outline of Grief Support Protocol

Purpose: ____

STEP 1 Lay the Foundation

_____ Prepare the physical environment.

_____ Stock client-education/support supplies.

_____ Assign/assume team member roles and responsibilities.

STEP 2 Implement Support Techniques

_____ Establish trust and rapport.

_____ Use a variety of appropriate verbal and nonverbal clinical communication skills and emotional support techniques.

_____ Provide clients with educational/support products, information, and referrals to take home. (These might include conversations/printed information about decisions to make prior to euthanasia, such as what to expect from the euthanasia procedure and body care options.)

STEP 3 Stay Connected through Follow-up Care

_____ Call clients within 24 hours to check on their well-being and clear up any questions or misunderstandings they might have.

_____ Send a handwritten condolence card or note as soon as possible.

_____ Schedule an appointment time if clients are picking up cremains and/or memorial pawprints. Ask if clients have questions or concerns they want to discuss.

_____ If case was unusual or especially emotional, debrief with team members; role-play and review case at weekly staff meeting to improve everyone's client-support knowledge and skills and personal ability to draw closure to patient loss.

Clinical Communication Skills

Nonverbal Communication

Only a small percentage of communication happens verbally. Along with *what* is said, communication is also *where* it is said, *how* it is said, *why* it is said, *when* it is said, *whom* it is said to, and what is *not* said. Nonverbal communication is conveyed through facial expressions, body postures, gestures, and hand movements as well as through writing, reading, and listening.

Nonverbal communication adds meaning to the verbal. For example, if a person who is crying tells you he or she feels sad, you not only believe him or her but probably also feel a great deal of empathy. The following nonverbal communication skills and techniques, used with verbal ones, enhance your message of compassion and care.

Structuring the Environment

Structuring the environment means paying attention to the various elements of your office, examination rooms, and consultation areas that can easily be moved and changed and arranging them to create the atmosphere you desire for your clients. For example, the way chairs and other furnishings in a room are placed can convey comfort, warmth, and understanding. The goal of structuring the environment is to invite your clients' emotions to arise, instead of shutting them down. You might place chairs so that conversations can take place face-to-face without barriers such as desks or examination tables between you and your clients. You might adapt examination rooms so that euthanasias can be performed on the examination table, on the floor, or even on a gurney rolled near the window so the pet and pet owner can be near the outdoors.

When anxiety is high, we all tend to become frozen into our positions. We forget we can stand up if we are sitting, walk around the room if we are standing, or even leave the room altogether if we need a few minutes to be alone. This rigidity can be overcome by a well-thought-out practice environment that allows for all of these options. Adapting the physical elements of your environment should therefore be a priority as you consider how to help your clients cope with grief.

Attending

Attending body language conveys that you are paying careful attention to the person who is talking to you. When your body posture is open, your eye contact is direct, and you are leaning slightly forward toward the speaker, you are demonstrating your availability and willingness to be of service. Attending behaviors include nonjudgmental facial expressions, encouraging gestures, affirmative head nods, and direct observation of what is occurring. You might get down on the same level with your clients by sitting if your client is sitting, or squatting to a child's eye level when greeting or talking to a child.

Active Listening

Active listening means listening for feelings rather than for the factual content of conversations. There is a difference between merely hearing someone and actively listening to what he or she is saying. Active listening incorporates paraphrasing, asking questions, and using attending behaviors such as making eye contact and using open body posture to encourage clients to say more.

Two minor, but important, nonverbal communication techniques inherent in the process of active listening are *necessary silences* and *minimal encouragers*. Necessary silences take place when you remain silent while others vent their feelings or gather their thoughts, rather than babbling to fill the silent, empty spaces. When emotions are high, it is tempting to babble in order to fill in these spaces; yet, remaining silent while others vent their feelings or gather their thoughts is often far more helpful. Minimal encouragers are simple responses that encourage people to continue talking. Minimal encouragers let people know you are an active participant in the communication going on between the two of you. They include head nods and phrases that indicate you are involved, such as "Uh, huh," "I see," and "For instance?"

Responding with Touch

Touch provides comfort, demonstrates care and concern, and often takes the place of reassuring words. It often has a calming effect and can help people slow their thoughts and steady themselves emotionally. There is some scientific evidence that touch affects the body physiologically, slowing heart rate and lowering blood pressure. Touch can be used to soothe a grieving client, to bring someone who is rambling back to the point, or to pull someone who has drifted away back to the present.

When using touch with clients, limit it to neutral or safe areas such as the shoulders and arms. Areas of the body that are not viewed as neutral or safe include the neck, hands, torso, lower back, and legs. In general, people dislike being patted on their backs or heads. This behavior connotes a sense of superiority on your part and can be viewed as condescending. If touching or hugging clients makes you uncomfortable, a substitute technique is to touch your clients' companion animals with care. Pet owners often judge your sensitivity based on how you handle their pets.

Demonstrations

Demonstrations are a way to simplify and to "walk clients through" medical information or procedures. Verbal descriptions generally accompany demonstrations. When used together, verbal descriptions and demonstrations give clients a step-by-step account of what needs to be done for their companion animal.

Demonstrations might include the proper way to bandage a wound or give medicine to a cat. It might consist of practice sessions with a syringe and an orange so clients feel more confident about giving their pets injections. Tours of your surgery suite or recovery room might also be considered a demonstration, especially when you explain the various procedures that will be done while your client's pet is in each room.

When clients have a visual understanding of what certain treatments entail, it is often easier for them to decide whether those options are right for them and their pet. Videotapes and DVDs demonstrating the key points of a treatment or surgical procedure can also aid in clients' decision-making process.

Written Information

The *written information* you provide to clients is another form of nonverbal communication. Much of the medical jargon and information familiar to you is very foreign-sounding and unfamiliar to average pet owners. Therefore, it helps to write things down or to draw pictures for clients. Drawings and written materials also allow clients to take information home so they can describe their pet's situation accurately and in full detail to the other members of their family.

Verbal Communication

Verbal skills make use of the spoken word. When using verbal skills, it's important to pay attention to your tone of voice and the pacing of your speech, because these have great influence on the meaning of your words. For instance, if you use the appropriate words to describe a situation but say them at a very fast pace, you may be viewed as feeling rushed, acting nervous, or being just plain insensitive, even if that isn't the truth about you. If you speak the same words too slowly, though, you may be viewed as dull or condescending. Monitor your voice tone when you are working with clients who are grieving. Words that are spoken softly and at a slightly slower pace than normal are usually viewed as more comforting than louder, more fast-paced speech.

To effectively convey your message of compassion and care, use the following verbal communication skills and techniques along with the nonverbal ones described above.

Acknowledging

Acknowledging is recognizing the existence or truth of something. It encourages people to deal openly and honestly with the emotions inside of them and with the reality of the situation at hand. You might say, for example, "I know you loved Ruby very much and that her death is very painful for you." Using this technique helps your clients acknowledge their own feelings about a situation.

Normalizing

Normalizing is lending credibility to others' thoughts, feelings, behaviors, and experiences by letting them know that their responses are normal. The symptoms of grief can seem quite disturbing when they are not clearly understood. Inform clients that it is normal for a wide range of emotions to accompany loss. You might say, "Your tears honor your special relationship with Ruby. You two were together for 10 years and were best friends. It's normal to miss her."

Giving Permission

Giving permission means encouraging clients to think, feel, and behave however they need to (within safe limits) without fear of judgment. This technique also allows clients to ask for what they want or to make requests that are important to them. For instance, before euthanasia, clients may ask for a soft blanket or floor pad to lay their animal on, to be able to feed their pet one last time, or to be present when their pet dies. You might say, "You and Ruby have shared a lot throughout your lives together. What else would you like to do for her as we plan for this difficult day?"

Asking Appropriate Questions

Asking appropriate questions helps you gather valuable information about the circumstances surrounding your clients' loss. Failure to ask clients questions can lead to problems; there are many consequences to making assumptions about your clients' needs.

The most helpful questions are open-ended, not closed-ended. A closed-ended question can be responded to with "yes," "no," "fine," or some other one- or two-word answer. Open-ended questions elicit more detailed information and create opportunities for clients to tell you more about what they are experiencing. Open-ended questions begin with "how" or "what" rather than with "why." "How" and "what" questions elicit thoughtful explanations. You might say, for example, "How will you know when Ruby is no longer enjoying life?" Questions that begin with "why" often elicit "I don't know" answers. "Why" questions also have a tendency to put clients on the defensive, making them feel they need to explain themselves to you. One word of caution: A well-placed, open-ended question can launch a lengthy client monologue, so use this technique only when you have adequate time to spend with clients.

Paraphrasing

Paraphrasing is the restatement or summary of clients' communication in order to test your understanding of their comments. When you paraphrase clients' comments, it reassures them that the intended message got through. It also provides clients with the opportunity to clarify what was meant if your understanding is inaccurate.

When paraphrasing words and emotions, it is also important to attend to your voice tone and pacing. For example, if a client is complaining loudly, you might offer an immediate response in an equally firm tone of voice, confirming that you understand there is a problem. Then, you can quickly move your client to a private room where you can attempt to alter his or her emotional level and gain some control over the situation by lowering your voice and slowing down your pace. Doing so will, in turn, slow down your client's side of the conversation and create an atmosphere more conducive to mutual listening and problem solving.

There are many ways to paraphrase. Easy ways to begin paraphrase statements are "It seems as though . . . ," "It sounds like . . . ," and "If I hear you correctly, you feel . . ." A final way to use paraphrasing is to summarize the main points of a lengthy conversation to ensure that you've understood your client's concerns. If your client says, "I don't know what I will do if Ruby dies while I'm not home. I'll never forgive myself," you might say, "It seems like you're worried that she'll die without you, and you'll feel guilty." Paraphrasing serves many purposes: It can help clients identify their own feelings or understand a dilemma, let them know that you are listening and that you understand what they are going through, encourage them to share, or enable them to work toward closure or to make a difficult decision.

Self-Disclosure

Self-disclosing is *briefly* sharing a personal experience when it may be appropriate and of use to clients. Self-disclosing about your own experiences with companion-animal death can help your clients feel less alone in their grief. When using self-disclosure, it is very important not to shift the focus away from your client and onto yourself. You might say, "I've lost pets to cancer, too, and I understand how difficult it is to say this final good-bye."

Gentle Confrontation

Gentle confrontation can be used to point out discrepancies or inconsistencies in what clients have said or done. It can also be used to set limits on clients' behaviors or expectations. Gentle confrontation may take the form of a question or a statement. For example, "You've been bringing Ruby to me for almost four years and, together, we've helped her through many medical problems. I can hear your disappointment about her failing condition, but I have to wonder if the anger you're expressing is really more about the failure of her latest treatment than about the quality of care she is receiving here."

Clients in need, or those who are upset, angry, or grieving, are often demanding and difficult to understand. They are prone to losing perspective. Because of their strong emotions, they may behave in ways in which they would not otherwise dream of behaving. Gentle confrontation can be a good communication technique because it can help you "stand up for yourself" without becoming defensive. With it you can sensitively, but firmly, help clients understand your own limitations, as well as the established policies of your practice. For example, you can say something like "I can see that you are disappointed that you can't stay with Nugget overnight. I know this is frustrating for you. I feel I have been clear with you regarding our policy that prevents clients from spending the night in our clinic. I wish it could be different for you, but I want to honor my clinic's decision."

Gentle confrontation may also be used to narrow the content of clients' conversation. Some clients ramble on about topics unrelated to animal care, making it difficult for you to cover pertinent topics with them. Clients sometimes steer conversations off track because they don't want to make difficult decisions or hear what you have to say. Gentle confrontation allows you to redirect these conversations and keep them on course. Begin with a comment on the subject the client has brought up, and then redirect to the subject you wish to pursue: "It would be easy for us to spend our time together discussing your son's upcoming wedding. Yet, we're meeting today to talk about what's best for Ruby. It may be time for us to make a plan for her end-of-life care."

Immediacy

Immediacy combines gentle confrontation and self-disclosure. The purpose of immediacy is to comment on the unspoken feelings or thoughts that exist in an interpersonal relationship. The use of immediacy requires you to talk openly with your clients about what you are feeling or experiencing *right now*. It is an extremely important skill for almost any difficult situation because it allows you to be honest with the other person about your feelings. For example, you might say: "Sharon, you seem upset with me. Did something I said offend or hurt you in some way?" Another example would be "Mrs. Watson, I would like to work with you to help Ruby. It would be helpful to me if you would share any concerns you might have so we can move forward from here."

This technique is most effective when used in a well-established relationship. You are commenting directly on the client's thoughts, emotions, and behaviors, and a new client may feel intimidated, exposed, or judged by this. If the technique is used too soon or too harshly, clients may react defensively.

E-mail, Telephone, and Social Media Conversations

The techniques described in this book are intended to be used during face-to-face interactions. We understand that e-mail, text messaging, Facebook, Twitter, and telephone conversations can also be powerful communication tools when used by skilled communicators. However, they can also lead to misunderstandings, as the visual cues that people rely on for accurate interpretation of words are missing. When using e-mail, text messaging, the telephone, or any other social media, keep the following points in mind.

When using the telephone, remember that your voice is your most powerful tool. Pay special attention to the tone and pitch of your voice and the pacing of your words. In addition, prepare yourself for potentially emotional calls by finding a quiet, controlled environment where you won't be distracted or interrupted.

Do not convey details about emotional topics, such as a pet's death, relapse, or body care arrangements, via e-mail, text message, social media message, or voice mail. Instead, ask your clients to call or visit you at your clinic.

Maintain your clients' confidentiality. If another family member or a coworker answers the telephone or returns your call, it may be best to refrain from providing him or her with the details of your patient's condition. Simply instruct the person who answers to ask your client to return your call. Of course, do not blog about the specific details of your cases. If you're a blogger or if you post updates about your professional life on Facebook or another social media site, remember that your clients may read these, too.

If clients have not returned your e-mail, text message, or call within a reasonable amount of time, try again. Messages get lost, and clients, especially emotional ones, sometimes forget to respond. It's your responsibility to make contact with your client and it is important that you keep trying until that task is accomplished.

Remember that when you contact clients during work hours, they may be unable to speak with you about emotional issues. The client may not have permission to take personal calls or the privacy needed to speak to you. If you do reach a client at work, tell him or her that you need to discuss a difficult issue and ask if it is a convenient time to talk. The client may prefer to arrange a telephone appointment for a time when he or she can speak more freely from a private area.

Give clients choices regarding the kind of information you will share with them in an e-mail or telephone call and how much detail to include before you proceed with these forms of communication. For example, on the telephone you might say, "I would be happy to explain the details of Misty's surgery to you. Would you like that information now?" It's best to ask rather than to overwhelm your client with information. One client may want to know everything immediately, whereas another will prefer to come in and see you face-to-face to hear the information.

A Financial Note on Clinical Communication

Your clients' age, gender, cultural heritage, religious orientation, and even political affiliation might influence how they behave, especially during emotionally charged interactions. These factors might also influence their beliefs about what is acceptable in terms of extensive medical treatments and end-of-life decisions for a pet. Keep in mind that, while the clinical communication skills and protocols described are effective with the majority of veterinary clients, individual differences must be considered.

SECTION TWO

Support Protocols for 14 Common Situations

SITUATION 1

Crises and Emergencies

Rhonda rushes her dog Romeo to your veterinary clinic on a Friday afternoon at 4:45 p.m. Romeo has just been attacked by another dog, his injuries are severe, and his life is in danger. Romeo needs immediate treatment, but Rhonda is clutching him to her chest and won't let you examine him. "My husband and son will be furious if they find out I left the door open when I was bringing the groceries in," she says. "I just wasn't paying attention! You have to fix Romeo! If he dies, they'll be devastated! This is all my fault . . . they'll both hate me forever!" By this time Rhonda is crying and, still cradling Romeo, she walks to the far side of the waiting room. But in a sudden burst of anger, she quickly returns to you and shoves Romeo into your arms, screaming, "Go fix him! Don't just stand there! Go fix him!" Then she collapses into a chair and sobs.

Assessment: What's Going On Here?

Rhonda is in crisis. Crises cause people to act in ways that are not normal for them. When people are in crisis, they may feel out of control, panicked, angry, and confused. They experience time as moving either very quickly or very slowly. Crisis makes it hard for people to listen and to later recall information.

People in crisis often display symptoms of shock and anxiety. Many are unable to think clearly or to follow directions. In the acute stage of crisis, some people behave in erratic or irrational ways. The skills and knowledge they normally use to cope with life are either forgotten or no longer work. Crises escalate when people feel helpless and cannot find effective ways to respond to events that are unfolding.

The purpose of providing client support during crisis is to direct people toward an acceptable resolution to their problem. Generally, the main goals in a crisis are to stabilize the situation and to stabilize your client.

Plan
Support Protocol: What to Say, What to Do

STEP 1 Lay the Foundation

- Designate one staff person (who is not involved in providing direct treatment for the animal) to facilitate your client's emotional support. This person should notify other clients about the emergency and reschedule their appointments, if necessary; wait with the client while the pet's medical condition is being evaluated, if possible; keep the client well informed about the pet's medical status while treatment is taking place; and offer the client tissues, a glass of water, and a telephone so he or she can notify other family members regarding the emergency.
- Structure the environment by gently, yet firmly, guiding the client to an office, an examination room, or even a treatment room, depending on the medical status of the animal. If the client insists on carrying the pet, allow this, place a firm arm around his or her shoulders, and quickly walk with the client and pet to wherever they need to go.
- Use touch and a soothing voice to calm the client.

STEP 2 Implement Support Techniques

- During a crisis, it is important to respond as quickly as possible and pay attention to what clients say they want and need, in addition to what you think they want and need. When clients feel that their needs are validated, they begin to relax and develop trust in you and are better able to listen to you and make decisions about the medical options you offer them.
- Acknowledge the client's emotions. Give permission to express them by saying, for example, "I see how much you love Romeo. I would expect you to cry in this situation."
- Clinical experience shows that clients who are deprived of contact with their ill or injured companion animal usually become more anxious and demanding. Everyone's needs are better served when clients are

invited and even encouraged to visit their pets while they are hospitalized. This is especially important if the prognosis is poor and the patient is not expected to live.

- If you are concerned about how clients may respond to seeing their pet hooked up to emergency equipment and monitors, take time to prepare them for what they will see. For most pet owners, the benefits of visiting a pet in critical condition or having the chance to say goodbye one last time far outweigh any anxiety about medical procedures or equipment.
- Occasionally someone other than the owner will bring an injured animal to your clinic. These animals have usually been injured without their owners' knowledge. If these "John Doe" animals have no identifying information, consider photographing them so that, if they die, they might later be identified.

STEP 3 Stay Connected through Follow-up Care

- When a crisis reaches a conclusion, make sure your client is calm and stable enough to drive home. It's difficult to function during a crisis, and even second-nature activities like driving can feel overwhelming for people. Sometimes it's best to encourage your client to call a friend or family member for a ride home.
- If you are sending the patient home with the client, provide written instructions about the pet's care and demonstrate any procedures the client might need to perform.
- When providing support during a crisis, it is important to assist your client with the situation at hand while at the same time assessing what his or her needs might be at a later time. For example, you may want to refer the client to community resources such as veterinary medical specialists or pet-loss support groups that can continue to provide assistance in the days and weeks ahead.
- As a veterinary professional, you will feel most successful when you are able to save the life of the animal brought to you during a medical emergency. Yet, this is not always possible. Even if your patient dies, however, you can provide top-notch care for the client. When your client thanks you for waiting with him or her, tells you that your frequent medical updates are appreciated, or simply lets you know that he or

she truly felt that you cared, you will know that your helping efforts made a difference in the client's emotional life. And the odds are in your favor that the client will return to your practice in the future.

ROLE-PLAY IDEAS

For hospital managers and client care specialists: Use the above situation to practice calming down a client in crisis. Pay attention to your voice, mannerisms, and nonverbal communication.

For veterinary technicians: Using the above situation, practice how you might provide periodic updates to the client. Practice your support techniques in trying to calm the client down.

For veterinarians: Practice working with a client using the above scenario. Pay attention to your voice tone, nonverbal communication, and responses to his or her anger, sadness, and shock. Practice providing periodic updates as to how the pet is doing, and practice making a referral for additional support.

Your Notes

SITUATION 2

Delivering Bad News

A client named Joanna rushes into your hospital holding her cat, Boots, in her arms. She is crying and distraught, and it's obvious that Boots is in respiratory distress. You immediately take the cat to an examination room and perform emergency care and 15 minutes of CPR. Despite all of your efforts, Boots dies. You must now meet with Joanna to deliver the bad news.

Assessment: What's Going On Here?

Joanna was clearly very upset by her cat's unexpected emergency, and she will most likely react in an emotional way when you deliver the news of the cat's death. Clients' reactions to bad news about their pet are often unpredictable, however. Therefore, when you deliver the news, be prepared to deal with a wide range of grief responses. Shock, disbelief, anger, blame, sadness, and even hysteria are common. Anxiety and shock may cause one client to appear calm, stoic, or too much in control. The client may say nothing but engage in intensive hand-wringing and aimless pacing. Anxiety may cause another client to smile or laugh inappropriately even when his or her pet has died.

Still other clients may react with rage, guilt, or confusion. They may sob, scream, and even hit or kick objects that are in the room. A few clients may accuse you of incompetence or even of making up a disease so you can charge them for expensive treatments. One or two may hang up on you if you're delivering bad news via the telephone or, when face-to-face, simply turn and walk out the door, leaving the pet behind.

Plan
Support Protocol: What to Say, What to Do

STEP 1 Lay the Foundation

- As in any other situation where you must communicate with grieving clients, you will need to make a plan that will allow you to communicate the information effectively.
- Think carefully ahead of time about where you would like to be with the client when delivering the bad news. Create a relaxed yet structured environment where you and your client can sit down, touch, and make direct eye contact.
- Stock a private area with tissues and arrange furniture in a way that allows you and the client to sit down and talk without a desk between you. This is often called a Client Comfort Room.
- Make sure the client has access to a telephone in case he or she does not have a cell phone on hand.
- Never deliver bad news in a public area or in front of other people. Delivering bad news is challenging enough without also having to deal with an audience.

STEP 2 Implement Support Techniques

- When delivering bad news, use a soft voice and speak more slowly than usual. Crisis intervention experts recommend creating a context of sensitivity and compassion. Provide the client with the basic facts and then listen and attend to his or her emotional responses without becoming defensive, guilty, or angry yourself. This is a tall order, but possible to accomplish if you understand the wide range of normal responses to grief. In most cases, when clients respond inappropriately to loss, they are not aware of how their words and behaviors may affect you. They are simply reacting. Later, when they realize what they have said or done, most clients who reacted in these ways feel embarrassed and apologetic. When you understand the grief process, you can normalize their behaviors and forgive grieving clients for taking their feelings about the situation out on you.
- When it's time to implement support techniques, try to predict how a client may feel about or respond to the news of the pet's death and then

proceed to offer information in brief, step-by-step conversations. Expect to deal with a wide range of grief responses, from angry accusations to complete silence. Be sure to use words such as "died" and "dead" so there can be no confusion in the client's mind about what has happened. It is not helpful to use euphemisms when discussing bad news.

- Deliver the bad news in four stages:
  1. Prepare yourself emotionally for the client's potential responses, keeping in mind that the client may be in shock. Reactions may include sadness, anger, crying, and denial.
  2. Tell the client that there is bad news that will be difficult to hear. For example: "Joanna, I have some difficult news that will be hard for you to hear." This prepares the client emotionally for what is to come.
  3. Proceed to offer the client information in brief, step-by-step increments, using clear and concise language. Offer information in slow, deliberate sentences, giving the client the opportunity to process what is being said before continuing to provide information. For example: "We did everything possible for Boots and performed CPR on him for 15 minutes. Despite our best efforts, we were unable to save him and he died. I'm so sorry."
  4. Give the client permission to express himself or herself by normalizing his or her feelings and using appropriate self-disclosure. Touch, attend, and paraphrase to deescalate tension and calm the client. Acknowledge your client's emotions, and do not take any comments that he or she makes at this time personally. For example: "I know this is a horrible shock for you and I can't imagine all you must be feeling right now. I want you to know that we want to support you in any way that we can." After a brief pause, you could continue with "Is there anything we can do for you right now? Would you like to call anyone, or would you rather have a little time alone for a few minutes?" If the client would just like some time alone, before you leave the room you could say, "We have some support materials for you when you feel ready."
- It takes time for most clients to fully realize the magnitude of what they have been told. Most will remember little about the first conversation they have with you and will have many questions later. If you are the

veterinary professional who delivers the news, it is important for you to proceed by asking the client what she or he needs next. For example, you can offer to provide more detailed medical information in an hour or so, either by calling or meeting with the client again, acknowledging that it is difficult to absorb information when first hearing that one's pet has died. You should also offer the client the option of viewing the pet's body.

STEP 3 Stay Connected through Follow-up Care

- Send a condolence card to the client and acknowledge how difficult it can be to lose a loved one (especially unexpectedly).
- Follow up with a phone call or another appointment if the client would so desire. This may be a perfect time to talk about how the client is dealing with things and find out whether he or she would like a referral for some extra support.
- Debrief with your staff, when possible, or make a note to discuss the situation at the next staff meeting or another appropriate time.

ROLE-PLAY IDEAS

For hospital managers and client care specialists: Practice delivering bad news using the above situation. Use the four-step process and seek feedback from your colleagues.

For veterinary technicians: Practice supporting a client while he or she is waiting for the doctor to deliver bad news about a pet's condition. Pay close attention to your verbal and nonverbal behavior.

For veterinarians: Using the above scenario, practice delivering bad news to a client. Use the four-step process, paying close attention to your verbal and nonverbal communication.

Your Notes ✍

SITUATION 3

Euthanasia Decision-Making

Dawn is sitting beside you in an exam room after a follow-up visit with her cairn terrier, Candy, who is terminally ill. You've told her that the prognosis is bad and it may be time to make end-of-life decisions. Biting her nails, she replies, "I don't know what I should do. I promised Candy I would always make the decision that was best for her, but I don't know what that is. I don't want to give up too soon if there is any chance for her to get better, but I don't want her to suffer either. If Candy were your dog, what would you do?"

Assessment: What's Going On Here?

Dawn's dilemma is not uncommon: Decision-making is one of the most difficult tasks that pet owners face. Whether the decision is fairly inconsequential (e.g., vaccinations, dental exams, diagnostic tests) or extremely serious (e.g., surgery, amputation, expensive treatments, euthanasia), many pet owners get stuck in the decision-making process and ask for additional guidance from veterinary team members. Yet, clients like the one who asked the question in the opening scenario are not just looking for a medical opinion; they are also looking for reassurance. They want to know that you will support them regardless of the decision they make.

But there is a problem with this situation. Most clients want to please the professionals with whom they work and hope to be viewed as cooperative, responsible clients. Thus, they may move ahead with the decision to euthanize based on your recommendation even if they are not yet ready to let go. Later, some of these clients may feel that you pressured them into euthanizing their animals. When clients believe their veterinarians rushed them through the process of saying goodbye and helping their pet die, it can cause irreparable damage to the veterinarian-client relationship.

Plan

Support Protocol: What to Say, What to Do

STEP 1 Lay the Foundation

- Structure the environment so there will be a quiet, calm space that allows for a potentially emotional conversation. Be sure to have plenty of tissues on hand. Pay attention to seating arrangements and always sit with clients rather than standing over them. Towering above clients or leaning on the door with a clipboard or case file pressed to your chest can be intimidating and make it very difficult for clients to speak openly about their feelings. When you sit with them without obstructions like a desk or table between you, you can be at eye level.
- Create an environment that will help the client make a decision. Brochures, pamphlets, and other resources should be readily accessible to provide guidance and inspire the client to start asking difficult yet necessary questions.

STEP 2 Implement Support Techniques

- Keep clients responsible for their own decisions. Rather than stating your personal opinion, you might say, "If Candy were my dog, I would be confused and upset, just like you are. Euthanasia is one of the most difficult decisions you will ever make in your life, and the fact is that you and I would probably be ready to face it at slightly different times. Even if I believe the time is right to help Candy die, you must also believe it, or it will be difficult for you to feel at peace with your decision." Another option might be "The truth is, Candy isn't my dog, and what I might do and what you might do could be very different. You are the expert on Candy. No matter what you decide, I'll support you and your decision."
- Acknowledge, validate, and normalize the difficulty of the client's decision.
- Use a variety of decision-making strategies to help clients make choices that are right for them and their companion animals. When handled

well, these stressful situations can actually improve or solidify your relationship with your clients. Following are some strategies to try:

- **Review the possible consequences.** Help your clients to think through every possible option so that they can make informed choices based on their preferred outcome. For example, you might say, "I know it's difficult to actually make an appointment to euthanize Candy, so let's talk about the options. While it's hard to schedule a time, if we do, we will know that we can create a peaceful death for Candy and give you the time you need to be with her. Or, we can wait and let nature take its course, hoping Candy will die more naturally at home, without experiencing a great deal of pain. There are a variety of things that could happen, though, if we wait. She could die while you are not home, or her pain might become more severe, and, as much as I'd want to be with you, I may not be available when you really need me. These are some points for you to think about. I know you will make the decision that is right for you."
- **Ask tough questions.** If the client still seems unable to make a decision, use attending behaviors and active listening skills to draw out his or her concerns. You may need to use immediacy and gentle confrontation to ask a few tough questions. These questions should be designed to help your client recognize the reality of the pet's situation. They are probing questions and must be asked without any judgment in your voice. Preface your questions with brief self-disclosure and a comment such as, "I am going to ask you something that is hard for me to say and may be difficult for you to hear." Then ask, "Are you telling yourself that this decision will be easier to make tomorrow or several days or weeks from now?" or "If you choose not to euthanize Candy, are you putting her needs ahead of your own, or are you putting your needs ahead of hers?" Be careful when you ask this last question. It must be asked very gently and with no judgment in your voice or in your facial expression.
- **Offer the illusion of choice and provide a back door.** In most cases, helping your clients make a small choice will direct them toward the outcome you desire, yet still give them some feeling of control. You could say, for example, "I know you've decided

to euthanize Candy, Dawn, but you're still struggling with when to schedule the procedure. For Candy's sake and with your agreement, I would like to make the appointment for tomorrow. Would two or four o'clock work best for you?" If your client becomes more anxious once she has committed to a course of action, you can conclude this technique by providing your client with a back door. A back door is a way to cancel her agreement. You could say, "If you find you simply can't go through with the procedure, Dawn, you can always change your mind and reschedule your appointment for another time."

- **Identify bottom lines.** A bottom line is a guideline by which your client can measure the factors that must be considered to make a decision. Bottom lines are different for everyone. When it comes to the decision about whether to euthanize a terminally ill pet, your client's bottom line might be her dog's inability to enjoy normal activities, her pet's level of pain and discomfort, the length of time her dog is expected to live, or even the cost of continuing to treat the animal. You might say, "Dawn, many pet owners find it helpful to imagine the circumstances that would need to arise for them to make this decision. I call this thinking about your bottom line. For some clients, the bottom line is the pet's inability to walk or to get up under her own power. For others, it's a change in the way the pet responds to them. Do you have an idea of what the bottom line might be for you and Candy?"
- **Enlist the pet's help.** When your client and his or her companion animal have a deep, special relationship, there is also a unique form of communication between them. When a decision regarding the pet's welfare needs to be made, you can encourage the client to enlist the pet's help so that the client doesn't feel he or she is making the decision alone. For instance, you could tell the client in this example, "Dawn, you and Candy have always had a special kind of communication. That hasn't changed. Even now, if you get down on the floor, lie beside Candy, and look into her eyes, she may, in a sense, tell you what she is feeling and what she wants you to do.

It's possible for the two of you together to make this decision about how and when we should help her die."

- **Help the client identify his or her own preferred decision-making techniques.** Different people make decisions in different ways. Some people are very logical and practical, for example, whereas others base decisions more on emotions. To help the client use these preferred techniques, you can say, "When you have faced really difficult decisions in your life, what have you done in the past to come up with a decision? You might try using those same skills right now."
- **Paint a picture regarding what the client will experience.** Many clients have never witnessed a pet's euthanasia and may have mistaken ideas about what actually happens during the procedure. With the client's permission, explain your protocol (see a detailed explanation in Situation 4) and tell the client that he or she can be present with the pet when it occurs. In other words, let clients know they will be able to hold or sit beside the pet, talk to the pet, and stroke the pet's head, ears, and so on while you perform your medical duties. Creating a comforting, peaceful vision of saying goodbye to a pet is often the key to facilitating that final decision.

STEP 3 Stay Connected through Follow-up Care

- Know that your client support efforts will be successful when your clients make decisions that are right for them and their companion animal, even though they may not always be the decisions *you* wish they would make.
- If the client has not yet reached a decision, provide printed information and referrals to other resources. These resources may be veterinary grief counselors, books, brochures, or websites (www.veterinarywisdomforpetparents.com, for example, can guide and prepare clients to face the loss of their pet).
- Once a client has made the decision to euthanize, make the appointment and notify your staff so the entire team can provide support as needed.

ROLE-PLAY IDEAS

For hospital managers and client care specialists: Using the above scenario, practice talking with a client who is struggling with a euthanasia decision and is pressuring you to say what you think he or she should do. Pay close attention to both your verbal and nonverbal communication. Are your body language and facial expressions inadvertently revealing what you think your client should do, rather than supporting your client's thoughts and feelings?

For veterinary technicians: Use the scenario to practice responding to the client's anxieties and questions. Since you provide nursing care, clients may be more likely to ask for your opinion over that of another staff person.

For veterinarians: Practice using both verbal and nonverbal communication to help a client like the one in the above scenario to make a decision about euthanasia. Be sure to practice a situation in which the client is resisting making a final choice. Practice responding to questions and emotions.

Your Notes

Client-Present Euthanasia

The Mathews family, including Sarah and Jeff; their 6-year-old son, Jonah; and their 13-year-old cocker spaniel named Buddy, arrive at the hospital. They are all holding on to each other for support, and Jonah also is holding a teddy bear. You have been expecting them for their client-present euthanasia visit and greet them at the door. They are hesitant to follow you into the back. You lead the way to the Client Comfort Room, where everything is set up for the euthanasia. As you invite the family to sit around Buddy, Sarah says she doesn't know if she can do this, and little Jonah starts crying.

Assessment: What's Going On Here?

The Mathews family was able to come to a decision about euthanizing Buddy, but they are having a hard time now that the moment has come, especially since they have planned to come into the room and be present when the procedure takes place. Today, most pet owners want to be with their companion animals when they die, and most veterinarians graciously accommodate their clients' wishes. But, like the Mathews family, clients need support at this time. Because the trend toward client-present euthanasia is so strong, it is essential that you develop euthanasia techniques and protocols that take into account not only the physical needs of your animal patients but also the psychological, emotional, and even spiritual needs of your human clients. Though traditionally, euthanasia procedures were performed in an impersonal, clinical way in order to protect both veterinarians and clients from painful emotions, today's euthanasia procedures are performed with technical skill and sensitivity, respect for clients' emotional needs, and compassionate support. Today, euthanasia represents one of the best opportunities you have to create a lasting bond with your clients.

Most veterinary practice teams view euthanasia as a professional privilege and as a gift that can be bestowed upon dying patients. Many companion animals are euthanized with their human family members in attendance in the context of a respectful and reverent ceremony. This compassionate act requires you to develop a deep understanding of the human-animal bond, the needs of grieving pet owners, and the components of a skilled and sensitive euthanasia technique.

In this modern model of euthanasia, euthanasia methods and possible side effects are thoroughly discussed with clients, and clients are involved in the choices and decisions pertaining to the process as much as possible. Clients are also supported after their pet's deaths has occurred.

Not all of your clients will want or require a lot of time or attention during their pet's euthanasia. Based on clinical experience, each client will make different choices. Some will choose total involvement and orchestrate a fairly complex euthanasia ceremony. Others will choose minimal involvement, opting for only a goodbye hug as they leave their animal with you. However, all clients will appreciate being given the option to be as actively involved as they choose to be in the euthanasia planning process and in the actual procedure.

Plan
Support Protocol: What to Say, What to Do

STEP 1 Lay the Foundation

- When the time is right, gently introduce the idea of euthanasia as soon as it is a viable medical option and offer it as one of the client's choices, along with further treatment, palliative and/or veterinary hospice care, and so on. Once the decision is made, clearly explain everything that will happen before, during, and after the procedure.
- Explain the emotional aspects, as well as the medical details, of the euthanasia procedure and give clients choices regarding their level of involvement in the death.
    - For example, you might say, "Mrs. Mathews, I know Buddy is very important to you and your family. Therefore, I am committed to

making his death as meaningful and as positive for you as possible. To decide whether or not you want to be with Buddy when he dies, you need accurate information about how I conduct euthanasia ceremonies. Would you like me to explain the procedures I use now?"

- ◦ With the owner's permission, you can continue with a step-by-step description of the medical details, while painting a comforting picture of how the client can be involved with the pet. For example, you might say, "While I do what I need to accomplish, you can pet or hold Buddy's head and paws. You can also talk to him, sing softly, or recite a poem or a prayer. In addition, you can play music, light a candle, or anything else that helps you. In other words, I want you to do whatever you need to do to feel you have said goodbye to Buddy in the most meaningful way possible."

- Help clients decide where their pet will be euthanized. For instance, if your clinic has a comfort room or outdoor garden area, show it to clients so they have a visual image of the comforting surroundings you can offer. If you have the staff and resources to offer home euthanasia, or if there is a veterinarian in your area who maintains a home euthanasia practice, let clients know about these options as well.
- On the day of the scheduled euthanasia appointment, when clients arrive for the euthanasia, don't leave them to sit in a busy waiting area. Instead, immediately take them to the agreed-upon euthanasia site. Be sure you have structured the environment that has been chosen so that you and your clients will have everything you need to cope with the pet's euthanasia. Stock tissues, client-support materials, clay pawprint kits, and scissors and small bags for fur clippings. If the euthanasia is to be performed on the floor, spread a large mat or blanket before clients arrive.
- Once your clients are settled, deal with logistical matters, such as signing consent forms, paying for the procedure, and making arrangements for body care, if they have not been settled already. It is best for these details to be taken care of prior to the actual procedure, if possible, or, even better, before the day of the euthanasia appointment. You do not want to be asking clients for payment after they have just been present at the death of a beloved pet.

- Before the euthanasia procedure takes place, give pet owners the opportunity to spend a short time alone with their companion animal, if they so desire. If clients feel rushed through the euthanasia process, this feeling can negate the other positive aspects of the experience. Be sure not to schedule back-to-back appointments requiring the same room.

STEP 2 Implement Support Techniques

- If clients have elected to be present, the use of a catheter is highly recommended. A catheter is not a sign that you doubt your own skill. The truth is that, even if you hit a vein 99 percent of the time, there are times when fate goes against you. If you have to poke several times for a vein, animals naturally begin to pull away from you. Clients often interpret this movement as their companion animal's way of struggling to stay alive. They may even feel that you are needlessly hurting their pet.
    - If you decide to use a catheter, the animal should be taken briefly to a treatment room and the catheter placed in the animal's rear leg. This placement allows clients to be near the pet's head while you are performing the procedure. If you are concerned about the added cost of using catheters for euthanasia, you can place nonsterile, previously used ones. You might explain this aspect of your technique by saying, "The first thing I will do to prepare for Buddy's euthanasia is to take him to the treatment area, shave a small area of fur on one of his rear legs, and place an intravenous catheter. The use of a catheter simply means that I can make the necessary injections more smoothly."
    - Sometimes the veins of very old or ill cats cannot be catheterized. If a deviation in technique occurs, it's important that you explain it to clients and prepare them for any consequences that may arise.
- Even though you may have already explained your euthanasia protocol to your clients during a decision-making consultation, review the steps again before you begin the procedure. During client-present euthanasia, it's not unusual to have friends and family members present who have not yet heard your description of what is about to happen. Reviewing the protocol allows everyone present to hold similar expectations.
- Over the past several decades, clinical experience has proven that, when clients are present, using a series of injections may be preferable to us-

ing a single euthanasia solution. This series most often includes (1) a saline flush to test the catheter; (2) a barbiturate, such as thiopental, to relax the animal; and (3) the euthanasia solution, usually pentobarbital sodium.

- Using a drug combination like this seems to minimize side effects, making the animal's death as peaceful and painless as possible.
  - Making three injections is another reason to use a catheter. You can explain why you are repeatedly injecting an animal by saying something like "The euthanasia method I prefer to use involves three injections. The first is a saline solution flush. This tells me that the catheter is working. The second is a barbiturate, which places Buddy in a soothing state of relaxation. The third injection is the euthanasia solution. This injection will actually stop Buddy's heart, brain activity, and other bodily functions, and ultimately cause his death. His death will take place within a matter of seconds."
- Even though this recommended euthanasia technique usually minimizes any possible side effects, they can still occur. Therefore, you should let the client know that these effects might be part of the euthanasia experience. You can do this by saying something like "You should also know that, although my technique is designed to eliminate them, there may be some side effects of the drugs. For instance, Buddy may urinate, defecate, twitch, or even sigh a bit after he dies. He will not be aware of any of this, though, and he will not feel any pain. In addition, Buddy's eyes will most likely remain open. Muscles close our eyes, and once death has occurred, Buddy will not have use of these muscles."
  - Before you begin the injections, tell the clients that you are about to begin and allow them time to say a final, heartfelt goodbye or to gather their pet in their arms. Keep in mind that anxiety is usually high just prior to and during euthanasia. Sometimes owners have momentary episodes of panic. If this happens, it is best for you to halt the procedure and attend to your client's emotions before continuing. You can say something like "This is always the most anxious and difficult moment, but we have all decided this is best for Buddy. Let's take a deep breath and say goodbye one more time." It goes without saying that, if clients become adamant about stopping

the procedure, it should be stopped, if it is still medically possible to do so. In the many years of our clinical experience, though, we have heard of very few practitioners who have ever encountered this situation.

- Once the procedure has begun, inject the drugs quickly, with little or no lapse of time between them. As they are injected, tell your clients what you are doing so they are kept abreast of how the procedure is progressing. For example, you might say, "I am injecting the first solution, the saline flush, to make sure the catheter I have inserted is working properly." Once that has been done, the next might be announced by saying, "Now I am giving Buddy a barbiturate that will make him sleepy and help him drift off and relax." When it is time for the last injection, you might say, "Now I am injecting the final drug."
    - Aside from these statements, it's best for you to remain silent. Most owners want to focus on saying goodbye to their animal and find comments, questions, and chatter distracting to their concentration.
- While you are injecting the animal, be discreet with needles and syringes. (Keep them in the pocket of a laboratory coat or a smock and return them there after each injection is completed.) The sight of needles causes great anxiety in some clients. Be sure they are not within reach of children who are present.
- This method of facilitating euthanasia usually goes so quickly and smoothly that most owners don't realize when their pets have actually died. It is important, then, to use a stethoscope to listen for a final heartbeat. This visible act reassures pet owners that their companion animal has truly died. After listening for a heartbeat, the animal should also be pronounced dead. You should do this by gaining direct eye contact with your client and stating in a clear, soft voice, "Buddy has died." Push yourself to use the word "died" or "dead," as euphemisms can be confusing for clients at this time. With your pronouncement, clients may gasp, cry, or sigh with relief. They may make remarks about how quickly death came and about how peaceful the experience was.
- Do not assume that owners of large animals do not wish to be present at their companion animal's euthanasia. The bond between humans

and their horses, llamas, or cattle, for example, can be as strong as the bonds humans share with smaller animals. While there are techniques you can use, such as catheter extension tubes or knock-down stalls, to minimize them, side effects are more common with large animals than with small ones. Their bodies may collapse suddenly to the ground, for example, or they may make involuntary movements or take agonal breaths after the death has occurred. Clients should be well informed about what they might witness and, once educated, should be allowed to choose their own level of involvement.

- After death has occurred, reassure the client about his or her decision to euthanize the animal. You might say, "Buddy's illness had gotten to the point where you could no longer help him medically. Helping him die peacefully and painlessly was the humane and correct thing to do. You prevented him from suffering needlessly." You can also express your own feelings of affection for the pet. For example, you might say, "I'm going to miss Buddy, too. He always wagged his tail for me." These statements may then prompt a spontaneous review of the pet's life, with pet owners sharing their special stories with you.
- After euthanasia, some clients want to leave the site quickly, while others need more time alone with their pet. Whenever possible, accommodate the client's needs. Don't assume that a client wants to be alone with the pet's body. Always ask your clients what they prefer.
    - If a client wishes to spend more time with his or her pet's body, this is a good time to make a clay pawprint, or even hoofprint, of the animal. When clients can take a personalized keepsake like this home with them, they may feel a bit better about leaving the pet's body behind with you. If clients wish to leave quickly, you can still make a pawprint and present it when they return to pick up the pet's cremains.

STEP 3 Stay Connected through Follow-up Care

- Contact clients the next day to see if they have questions or concerns about the way the pet died. The best indicator that you have been effective and sensitive is a satisfied and relieved client. Many clients who have been present at a pet's euthanasia make comments like "I feel sad that he's dead, but happy that we could give him such a gentle death,"

A Word about Veterinary Hospice Care and Home Euthanasia

Many pet owners struggle with the idea of euthanasia and prefer to keep their dying pet comfortable at home. If your clinic provides veterinary hospice care, or if there is a veterinary hospice program available in your town, this is a valuable option to offer your clients.

If you provide home euthanasia, be prepared to deal with strong emotions (clients often feel more comfortable expressing emotion when they are on their own "turf"). Remember to bring multiple quantities of everything you might need for the procedure so you won't be caught without something. Have a checklist to go through each time, and restock your home euthanasia kit as needed.

Offering home euthanasia requires you to expend more of your time and staff resources, so you should charge accordingly. Clients are usually understanding about the extra effort home euthanasia requires, and most are willing to pay more for the service. However, to avoid any misunderstandings, be sure to tell clients about your fees before you agree to perform home euthanasia.

and "I never knew that witnessing death could be so helpful. I feel like I can let go of him now, knowing he died so peacefully."

- Grateful clients often want to give something back to the veterinary professionals who helped them and their pet at such a crucial time. Thus, they send thank-you notes, gifts of appreciation, and donations to the practice. They also tell their friends about you. A noticeable boost in your business, due to a reputation for being sensitive and compassionate, is the ultimate success.
- Supporting grieving clients after their pet dies is just as important as supporting them before and during the procedure. Reaching out to clients via the mail, telephone, or in person is not only a sign of compassion but also a wise business practice.
- It is always best to ask for and process payment for a euthanasia at the same time that you schedule the appointment, even if it is several days ahead of the event. It can become difficult to ask for payment later on when the client is grieving the loss of the pet. If you do need to ask for payment on the day of the euthanasia itself, take care of the charges before the procedure begins so your client is free to handle the emo-

tional issues of the day during the procedure and after the pet's death has occurred.

The day after the euthanasia, a team member should call the client to express the team's condolences and to ask the client how he or she is doing. The team may also send a note expressing sympathy, signed in a personal way by any team members who know the client. But do not send an invoice with this note or mention the payment issue in this initial phone call. Just show the client that you care. The step of making a phone call or sending a note of sympathy should be taken regardless of whether payment has been received. Once this step has been taken, wait at least five business days before sending the euthanasia invoice.

After you have sent the invoice, if payment is not received after a week or two has passed, call the client again or send a follow-up invoice. The team member who makes this type of phone call should still begin with words of sympathy. For example, "Mrs. Johnson, all of us here at the pet hospital have been thinking about you during this difficult time. How are you doing?" After listening to her answer and responding to Mrs. Johnson in an empathetic way, the team member could say "It's not easy to ask you about this, but it has come to our attention that payment has not been received for your appointment. Will you be able to send payment? You can also stop by to make the payment in person. Everyone here would like to see you again. If you have any further questions for Dr. Richards, you could talk with her then. If it's more convenient for you, you can send the payment in, of course." Once arrangements have been made, be sure to say, "Thank you for understanding. We are all looking forward to seeing you" (or, if she prefers to mail the payment, "Thank you for understanding. We would still love to see you sometime if you are in the neighborhood and have time to stop by").

- Sometimes clients invite the veterinary practice team to their pet's funeral. Some funerals are simple, private ceremonies. Others are elaborate, public goodbye rituals, complete with casket and graveside service. You may want to attend some of these as a way for you to say goodbye to a special patient. This may be especially true if you conduct home euthanasias. Whether or not you choose to attend them is up to you, however. If you must decline a client's invitation, you might say something like

"Sarah, while I would like nothing more than to be able to attend the memorials of all my patients, I've found that attending these ceremonies simply takes me away from the clinic too much. I won't be able to join you and your family in person, but I will be with you in my heart. Buddy was very special to me, too, and all of us here will miss him."

ROLE-PLAY IDEAS

For hospital managers and client care specialists: Role-play a scenario in which you "check in" a client who has come to euthanize his or her pet. Practice supporting the client, taking the client and pet to a private room, talking about paperwork, and discussing body care issues. Make sure that the client knows what to expect. *Note: In many pet hospitals and clinics, the euthanasia protocol is such that the client care specialists and hospital managers are rarely present at the actual time of euthanasia. While they may not be involved in the actual procedure, it is still critical for them to understand and be familiar with all the things the client can expect. It's also important for them to make time to say their own goodbye to the patient and perhaps the client when it is time for the client to leave the hospital. If you work at a practice with more than one veterinarian, make sure that you are familiar with each doctor's euthanasia procedure.*

For veterinary technicians: Practice being relatively quiet with a client while he or she says goodbye to a pet following euthanasia. Although it may feel silly to do so, practice your support skills by using appropriate touch and tone of voice. Practice answering any questions that may have arisen in the client's mind about how the euthanasia unfolded. If your clinic makes clay pawprints or other keepsakes for clients, practice making these and presenting them to a client.

For veterinarians: Practice performing a euthanasia where something goes wrong medically (the catheter slips out, the dose of barbiturate is inadequate, etc.). Practice responding to these problems and talking the client through them.

Your Notes

SITUATION 5

Viewing Bodies

Your client Helen's long-haired dachshund, Pixie, just died during emergency surgery. You've given Helen the news. By now, she's calmed down a little from the initial shock and outpouring of grief. You know that she'll be better able to grieve if she sees Pixie one last time, but you also know that many clients are uncomfortable with the idea of seeing a pet's body or even afraid.

"Helen," you begin, "would you like to see Pixie's body and say goodbye?" Helen replies, "Oh, no, I couldn't. . . . No, I don't want to see Pixie like this." "Helen," you say, "I know that the thought of seeing Pixie's body is difficult, but I want to assure you that, in my experience, it usually helps people to see their pet and to have a chance to say goodbye."

Helen looks around the room, lost in thought. "Maybe I do want to see Pixie. It's just that the thought of it makes me nervous. I've never seen a dead body before."

Assessment: What's Going On Here?

Death seems very foreign to many people in our modern society. Unlike our ancestors, we do not often have open caskets at funerals. The bulk of our population is in urban areas where people are not used to the idea of animals dying. Therefore, death can seem frightening. It is no wonder that Helen is nervous about seeing Pixie's body. Many people say they would prefer to keep only the happy memories of their pet when he or she was alive and that they do not wish to see the pet after it has died.

This choice can be a problem, however. There is a strong correlation between viewing a beloved pet's body and the progression of normal, healthy grief. Grief experts agree that seeing a body helps people accept the reality of death. It also allows pet owners to say a heartfelt goodbye to their pet. Sometimes clients or other family members who were not present when a pet died do wish to view the animal's body before it is buried or cremated. This can be an emotionally healthy choice. If clients are hesitant, you can educate them about the benefits and offer this option again.

If a pet's body is going to be viewed after death, take time to prepare it so your clients will be comforted by the image they see. This means washing the pet's fur if it has been soiled, tucking the pet's tongue back into the mouth, and positioning or covering the body so the pet looks natural and at peace. Once you've prepared the pet's body, clients also can be prepared regarding how they might want to interact with the body. For instance, they can be encouraged to touch, hug, and even hold their pet.

In the example above, once Helen decides to see Pixie, the veterinary team member could say: "Now, before we go to Pixie, let me prepare you a bit for what you'll see and be able to do. When you see Pixie, her body will still be warm and her eyes will be open. Pixie is covered with a blanket from her head down, but you may remove it if you want to see her entire body. As you remember, there are stitches on Pixie's abdomen where we made the incision during surgery. It's all right for you to touch Pixie, to pet her, and even hold her if you want to. Even though we've done our best to clean her, her body may still be slightly soiled due to the release of her bowel and bladder. There is a brush and a scissors in the room if you want to groom her or clip some of her fur to take with you. And, if you want it, we can make a clay print of her paw for you to take home with you."

Also be sure to ask your clients if they want you to be present during the viewing. Some will want the company, whereas others will want to have a few minutes alone.

Plan
Support Protocol: What to Say, What to Do

STEP 1 Lay the Foundation

- Prepare a private room so clients can spend some time saying goodbye to their pets. If your clinic has a Client Comfort Room, this is an ideal environment for this activity. If clients are able to sit on the floor, you might want to place a large pad or blanket on the floor and then place the pet's body on top of it so clients can be as near to their pets as possible. If clients are not able to sit on the floor, prepare an exam table with a soft blanket or small pad. Place a chair nearby so clients can sit near their pet if they wish to spend some time.
- Before a client is allowed to view the pet's body, clean the body of any blood or waste material and position it in a pleasing way for the client to see. The body should be curled slightly, with the head and limbs tucked into a sleeplike position. This is most easily accomplished by placing the body in a container of some sort. Place it on a fleece blanket or soft pad within the container and cover the body from the neck down, leaving the face and head exposed so the client can see and talk to the pet.
    - Positioning a body is especially important if it is to be placed into a casket or other container for burial or transport at a later time, or if you are keeping the animal's body in a cooler until other family members can view it or pick it up. If animals, particularly large dogs, are allowed to stiffen without being curled into a sleeplike position, placing them in a casket or even on the backseat of a car is nearly impossible. For this reason, it's a good idea to keep a box, a vinyl casket, or another container at your clinic for viewing and storage purposes.

STEP 2 Implement Support Techniques

- Acknowledge and normalize the client's anxiety. You might say, "I know that the thought of seeing Pixie's body is difficult." This may also be the time to provide brief education about the benefits of seeing a loved one's body. You might say, "Helen, in my experience, it can be comforting, in the long run, if you say goodbye and see for yourself, beyond the shadow of a doubt, that Pixie has died. It's always your choice, but many of my clients find they have regrets later if they don't take a final moment to be with their pet."

- Don't assume that a client would like time alone with a pet unless the client agrees to it. (Never lead a client into the room where the pet's body is without asking and then preparing the client.) Once the client seems comfortable viewing and touching the body, ask again if he or she would like some time alone.
- Give the client permission to touch, hold, and talk to the pet.
- Lead the way to the examination room or visitation site. If the client wishes to have some time alone, leave the room and tell the client how soon you plan to return. If the client asks you to accompany him or her during the viewing of the body, make the first move toward touching, petting, and talking to the animal. This is a prime time to act as a role model for the client so he or she will have a better idea of what to do. You may have to reiterate your verbal permission for the client to touch or hold the pet (depending upon the condition of the pet's body). Holding a pet's body after death is not abnormal or morose and you should offer this choice to your clients whenever possible. In fact, grief experts who work with parents whose child has died of Sudden Infant Death Syndrome encourage the parents to hold, rock, and even sing to the baby before the baby's body is taken away. These final acts of love can be extremely helpful with the grief process to follow.
- If your clinic makes clay pawprints or other keepsakes for clients, ask the client if he or she would like to help you make one. This activity can provide a welcome focus for the visit and create a much-appreciated link to the pet, as well as a positive connection to you and your clinic after your client goes home.
- If the client is not taking the pet's body with him or her after viewing it, you or another staff member should stay with the animal's body at the viewing site. Often owners will take one last look back at the pet before actually leaving. When they see a familiar face next to the pet, they feel reassured that their companion animal's body will not be forgotten or treated with disrespect once they leave.

STEP 3 Stay Connected through Follow-up Care

- When clients have been well prepared to view a pet's body and have been given the time to say a private, personal goodbye, they will almost always thank you. Even though anticipating a viewing often creates anxiety, the actual viewing of a body usually provides relief. Creating the opportunity to view a beloved pet's body and offering clients the choice to do so is an extremely effective way to provide grief support.
- Send a condolence card or follow-up letter that arrives within a few days, and make a phone call to the client within 24 hours to answer any questions or provide further assistance, if needed. These are important and very meaningful gestures in any grief situation.

Offering Condolences

Offering condolences and creating keepsakes are standard practices in most veterinary clinics today. Reaching out to clients after their pet dies is not only a sign of compassion, it is also a wise business practice. For one reason or another, a significant number of clients do not return to a veterinary practice after their pet dies. However, a friendly, concerned contact after the death of a pet can break through this avoidance and denial aspect of grief and reassure clients that you understand their loss and will welcome them back at any time. The vast majority of pet owners do not view condolences and memorials as morbid, intrusive, silly, or overly sentimental. They view them as sensitive ways for you to honor the deep, special bond they shared with their companion animal.

If an after-death conversation is taking place in a public area (the grocery store or your clinic's waiting room), structure the environment by inviting your client to join you in a more private place (such as a coffee shop next door to the store or your office). You might say, "Jill, it sounds like it might feel good for you to talk a bit about CeeCee, and I'd like to hear more about how you've been. Do you have time for a cup of coffee over in the deli?"

While you are offering your condolences, you can also invite clients to contact you if they have further questions or concerns. By taking advantage of the opportunity to educate clients about normal grief, you are doing them a great service. If you're sending a condolence card or note, include printed grief education materials and referrals to local pet-loss support groups or pet-loss counselors.

Condolence cards and telephone calls should be sent or made as soon after a pet's death as possible. Whether you're writing or speaking the words, recall something unique about the pet and refer to it in specific terms. For example, you might say, "I'll always remember CeeCee's pretty blue eyes and the long, sweet looks she would

continues

Offering Condolences, continued

give us." This reassures clients that you are reaching out to them personally and not treating their case as just another statistic.

Verbally acknowledge the pet's death during the first face-to-face, post-death contact you have with your client, even if this is several months after the death in a public place like the grocery store. Use direct eye contact, a quiet voice, and touch (if it seems appropriate) and say something like "Hello, Jill. I haven't seen you since CeeCee died. How have you and your family been since then?"

If your client begins to cry at the mention of her pet's name, normalize her tears and give her permission to cry and to talk about her pet and her feelings of grief. Remember, tears are normal and nothing to be ashamed of. Attend, paraphrase, listen actively, and, if appropriate, self-disclose about your own need to talk and to cry after a pet you loved died. Encourage your client to find a way to memorialize her pet if she hasn't already done so.

Most pet owners find it meaningful to have an object that links them to their pet. This object may be a dog's collar, a cat's toy mouse, a special blanket, or even a food dish. The object may also be part of the actual animal, such as a feather, the wool of a llama, part of a horse's mane or tail, or a pawprint set in clay. Remind clients that if these objects comfort them, they may keep them with them or in plain view in their home, rather than stuck away in a box or drawer.

Just as there are many ways to offer your condolences to clients, there are many ways you can help clients memorialize their pet. For instance, you can send flowers or make donations to animal organizations or to special service groups in the name of your clients' pet. You can make clay prints of the pet's paws, and you can give clients permission to create their own memorials. Many pet owners collect their memories into a scrapbook or photo album or on videotape.

Here is a sample condolence letter:

Dear John, Jill, and Meghan,

I have thought of you so often since CeeCee died. I want you to know that I believe your decision to help her die was the right one. Her cancer had advanced to the point that her quality of life was greatly diminished, and she just wasn't enjoying life much anymore. During treatment, you did everything you could for her and, in the end, spared her any further pain and suffering.

Our staff made a donation to the local humane society in your sweet CeeCee's name. I remember you said you adopted her there twelve years ago. We also hope CeeCee's collar and the clay print we made of her paw are comforting keepsakes for you. It can be comforting to keep familiar mementos from our pets' lives.

The next few days and weeks are bound to be sad for you all. I've included enclosure cards that provide helpful information about grief and about supporting children through this time. As I said when we spoke yesterday, we care about you and want you to let us know if we can be of any further support to you.

Sincerely,

Jean Wills, DVM, and Your Friends at Animal Care Hospital

ROLE-PLAY IDEAS

For hospital managers and client care specialists: Practice the above scenario and talk with the hypothetical client Helen about what it might be like to view Pixie's body. Discuss reasons why this might be helpful and then accompany Helen into the viewing room. Practice offering support while Helen holds Pixie. Be sure you have prepared the body for viewing prior to Helen's visit. Does your clinic keep appropriate containers on hand to accommodate this?

For veterinary technicians: Using the above situation, practice attending, paraphrasing, and active listening while you support Helen's grief and address her questions and anxieties. Practice asking Helen if she would like to help you make a clay pawprint or other keepsake of her pet and then practice making that memento with her.

For veterinarians: Practice the scenario above, providing the necessary education and support. Additionally, have a detailed discussion with the entire staff about the physical as well as emotional logistics involved when a pet owner wishes to view a body. Talk about all the specifics that may be involved, such as cleaning up blood, suturing wounds, brushing the pet's hair, using blankets, and so on. (This discussion can also be coordinated by the hospital manager.)

Your Notes ✍

SITUATION 6

Grief Responses to Pet Loss

One of your clients, Mary, sits in your exam room crying softly as you talk to her. You've just given her the news that her Basset hound, Freddie, has cancer. Now you're providing her with the information she needs to take the next steps. You say, "Should I give you a minute, Mary?" She replies, "No, I'm okay. I'm listening. . . . I'm sorry I'm crying. Freddie is still alive, so I shouldn't be crying."

Assessment: What's Going On Here?

As human beings, we are meant to grieve before, during, and after the death of a loved one. It is a normal, natural, spontaneous, and *necessary* emotional process. Mary in the example above is experiencing the very common phenomenon called *anticipatory grief.* She is also experiencing the common phenomenon of being embarrassed about expressing her emotions. In this section we will deal primarily with the issue of emotional grief responses such as crying.

People express their grief in many ways, but typical grieving often includes crying. People cry when they are grieving because it is a natural reaction to pain. Crying is an effective way to release emotion and an essential part of the grieving process. Still, like Mary in the opening dialogue, many people feel embarrassed or ashamed of their crying and view it as an emotional outburst or a sign of weakness. Dr. William Frey, a biochemist and leading authority on human tears, has noted that "people have the right to be human, to feel, to cry. They need to know there is no need to deprive themselves of the natural, healthy, release of emotional tears."

One of the biggest obstacles to helping others when they cry is the fear that you will cry, too. For this reason, you might find yourself wanting to avoid clients who are upset or even discouraging clients from being present at their pet's euthanasia. The fear is that, if you are upset, you won't know what to say or what to do to help your grieving clients. Yet, clients rarely report that they disliked it when a veterinarian or staff member cried. In fact, it touches clients deeply when you cry with them.

People generally feel better after crying. In general, studies have found that people with supportive friends and family who encourage them to cry are healthier than those who experience less encouragement from others to cry and to discuss their feelings of grief. It follows, then, that the best way you can support your crying clients is to encourage them to "get it out." Support them while they sniffle, sob, or wail. If clients exhibit extreme displays of emotion, such as uncontrollable sobbing or a panic attack, help them work through their waves of emotion. Never leave the room because you assume your clients want to be alone. The act of leaving the room may signal your own embarrassment or disapproval of their grief. All forms of crying are healthy and acceptable. Your job when providing client support is to become comfortable with tears.

Before providing support, prepare yourself to deal with a wide range of expressions of grief, including tears, anger, guilt, depression, and even stoicism, flippancy, and relief.

Plan
Support Protocol: What to Say, What to Do

STEP 1 Lay the Foundation

- Whether you are talking with a client whose pet has died or one whose pet is fatally ill or severely injured, structure the environment in a way that invites and supports the expression of emotion. For example, take the client to a private, comfortable room with soft lighting that provides privacy.
- Give the client permission to cry. Offer him or her a tissue and a place to sit down, saying, "Take your time and let it out, Mary. I'm right here if you need me." It's essential always to have a box of tissues in the room. This is one of the most powerful types of nonverbal communi-

cation in supporting grief. The presence of tissues tells the client loud and clear that it's okay to cry and to grieve without feeling that he or she has to keep up a conversation with you.

STEP 2 Implement Support Techniques

- Acknowledge your client's emotional expression of grief. You might say, for example, "I can see how sad [or angry, etc.] you are about Freddie's diagnosis."
- Normalize your client's tears and emotions. You might say, "I would expect you to cry and be upset in a situation like this."
- Touch your client lightly on the arm or shoulder or give the client a hug, if you sense that providing nonverbal comfort is appropriate.
- Self-disclose by crying yourself if you're moved to do so. Crying demonstrates compassion and shows empathy for your client and his or her pet. If you cry easily, you might say, "I often cry during times like this. I can still do my job, though, and be here for you."
- When possible, respect your client's need to end the conversation or leave your clinic quickly. It can be extremely uncomfortable for some people to show emotions like anger or sadness in public. These clients may feel an urgent need for privacy, especially if they feel they need to cry. Other clients may feel flooded by strong emotions when they hear sad news and need time alone to clear their head before continuing the conversation with you. In situations like these, it's not uncommon for clients to attempt to end the interaction that was taking place between you, either by shutting down completely (showing no emotion at all and even being unable to speak) or by suddenly talking a lot and even using inappropriate humor to comment on the situation.
- If the client expresses his or her grief through anger, it is important to understand what is driving that anger and not to become too defensive. Most people who display anger with their grief do so in very short bursts and without any real desire to hurt anyone. If you spend time acknowledging their grief, the anger usually lessens, especially if you use immediacy and make them aware of it. For example, you might say, "Mary, I can hear in your voice how angry you feel about Freddie's death and I would also imagine that you are feeling terribly sad. There's nothing fair about this situation and I'm sorry that you have to go through it."

    - If a client's anger appears to be over the top and you feel threatened, it is necessary for you to set boundaries to protect yourself and your staff. If a client refuses to work with you or becomes inappropriate with his or her anger, you should tell the client to leave and not return and that you will contact the police, if necessary. Your responsibility to support your client does not supersede your responsibility to ensure a safe working environment.

STEP 3 Stay Connected through Follow-up Care

- Remember that two responses will tell you that your clients appreciate the grief support you provided. They will return to your practice when they are ready to treat their pet, or they will call or write you to thank you for your kindness after a pet has died. In short, when you provide high-quality grief support, your professional relationship is likely to continue with an even deeper feeling of mutual care and loyalty.
- Check-in telephone calls should be made as soon after a pet's diagnosis as possible. During the call, invite the client to contact you with any further questions or concerns and take advantage of the opportunity to educate him or her about normal anticipatory grief. If you speak with the client in person, provide printed materials about decision-making and preparing for pet loss, along with referrals to local pet-loss support groups, pet-loss counselors, or online resources.
- Some pet owners find it meaningful to have an object that links them to their pet. This object may be a dog's collar, a cat's toy mouse, a special blanket, or even a food dish. The object may also be part of the actual animal, such as a feather, the wool of a llama, part of a horse's mane or tail, or a pawprint set in clay. It's helpful to reassure clients that, if these objects comfort them, they can be kept in a special place in their home, rather than stuck away in a box or a drawer.

ROLE-PLAY IDEAS

For hospital managers and client care specialists: Use the opening scenario to practice supporting a client who is crying. You may need to dig a little to get connected with these strong emotions. Practice normalizing the client's tears. Remember to pay attention to your tone of voice while using the verbal communication skills you will need in this situation.

For veterinary technicians: Practice supporting a client who has just heard bad news about a beloved pet and begins to cry. Normalize his or her emotions and respond to the client's apologies for being upset.

For veterinarians: Practice supporting a client who is grieving the news of a pet's terminal illness. Respond to the client's tears, paying attention to your tone of voice, your word choice, and your demeanor. Also practice supporting a client who expresses other strong emotions, such as anger or depression, and consider how you would provide nonjudgmental and nondefensive support. Practice making a referral for additional grief support.

Your Notes

SITUATION 7

Handling Body Care Options

Berkley, a nine-year-old yellow lab, underwent exploratory surgery. During the procedure, Berkley was found to have cancer all through his abdomen. The veterinarian contacted Berkley's owners, Jim and Marge, and together they decided to euthanize Berkley while he was still anesthetized. Jim and Marge told the veterinarian that they would like to have their dog's body back for burial.

Thinking that his clients would probably not want to see their pet after death, the veterinarian placed Berkley in a large, black plastic bag and sealed it tightly with a twist tie. When the clients arrived an hour later to pick up Berkley's body and were given the bag, they were confused. They believed their dog had been too big to fit into the bag that was lying in front of them on the floor of the examination room. Reluctantly, they removed the tie and looked inside. At that point they saw what had been their big, cuddly dog stuffed into a garbage bag, contorted into a grotesque posture. Crying, the clients struggled to carry their dog's body out to their car and left without even talking to the veterinarian.

When the veterinarian was told that his clients had left abruptly, he felt confused and a bit angry. He thought he had done what his clients had asked him to do and had handled the body in the way he thought would be best for them. He didn't understand their reaction.

Assessment: What's Going On Here?

Care of a pet's body following death is a delicate issue in terms of the client/veterinary professional relationship. Since many owners have invested many years, much love, and a substantial amount of money in the physical care of their companion animals, their pet's body remains important to them even after death. When clients perceive that their pet's body has not been treated with respect and reverence, their grief is often exacerbated, and the relationship with their veterinarian severely jeopardized.

This is what we see in the example above. The clients knew their dog was being euthanized, but they assumed that the body would be treated respectfully. The veterinarian, however, did not realize how important this issue can be to clients. The mismatch between client expectations and reality caused a major breach in the relationship. More important, the veterinarian missed an opportunity to help his clients with the grieving process and probably made the situation even more painful for them.

It's sometimes tempting to judge your clients' body care decisions. For example, there are clients who choose to have their horse cremated, spending thousands of dollars to do so. Others bury their companion animal in an expensive casket similar to those used for humans, or even hire taxidermists to preserve their pet's body so it retains the same appearance after death that it had in life. When it comes to body care, the measure of success is not whether your clients make the body care decision that *you* believe is right, practical, moral, or even sane. Rather, success is achieved when you facilitate honest, open, nonjudgmental discussions about body care and help your clients arrive at decisions that are *right for them*. These are the body care decisions that bring both you and your clients peace of mind.

Plan

Support Protocol: What to Say, What to Do

STEP 1 Lay the Foundation

- Whenever possible, help clients make decisions about body care prior to the death of a companion animal. Owners should be offered all the body care options that are available to them, and each option should be explained honestly and in a sensitive manner. The cost of each option should also be disclosed. If bringing up the topic of body care causes your own anxiety level to rise, say something like "This subject is always difficult for me to talk about, but I need to know what you would like to do with Berkley's body." It's wiser to reveal your own vulnerabilities than to make hurtful assumptions regarding your clients' wishes.

- Explain body care options in a private area. Use a conversational, quiet voice and respond to your clients' tears or questions with touch, attending behaviors, and honesty. When discussing body care options, you might say, "Jim and Marge, I can offer you three options for taking care of Berkley's body after he dies. The first option is for you to take him with you and bury him in a pet cemetery or in an appropriate place on your own property. If that is your choice, we encourage you to bring something like a blanket or a nice box from home to transport his body in, because our options here are limited to large plastic bags or vinyl caskets, which cost between thirty and fifty dollars. Second, you can cremate Berkley's body and either keep his cremains, dispose of them yourself, or ask the crematory to dispose of them for you. If you want the crematory to return them to you, and you decide to keep them rather than scatter them outdoors, you may wish to choose an urn or another kind of container to keep them in. Cremation has become a popular and practical body care option for pets because so many people in our society move quite often. This way, you can always take your pet with you. Your third option is to have us take care of Berkley's body for you. Although I wish I had a more pleasing option to offer you, my only option is [mass incineration, mass burial at the local landfill, or delivery to a rendering company—fill in the blank with whatever is accurate for your area]."
    - Since the majority of mass burials take place in landfills, clients should be given this information. Though it might not matter to some of your clients, the thought of burying their companion animal at a landfill might be quite distasteful to others.
- Use visual aids, along with demonstration and written information, during this explanation. For example, if your practice is able to make caskets or urns available for owners to purchase, samples and pricing can be shown. You can also offer to show your clients what the cremains of a dog or a cat look like. Many people think cremains are like

the gray, papery ashes that remain in a fireplace after a log has been burned, but they are actually more like sand or small pebbles, often with larger chips of bone included.

- Body care options also sometimes need to be explained to children. It's helpful to draw pictures and use appropriate props such as caskets, urns, and cremains to explain the concepts to kids. Think ahead about how you will explain these options to children, and make sure the parents approve of including the children in the discussion ahead of time. Some parents like to shield children from these matters, but when it is done with sensitivity, including children in these talks is often helpful to them.

STEP 2 Implement Support Techniques

- Normalize body care choices. A pet owner may feel foolish about his or her desire to bury or cremate a pet, particularly if the companion animal is large (e.g., a horse or llama) and doing so is very expensive. Burial and cremation of animals are becoming more common all the time, however, and there is no reason a client should feel embarrassed about making one of these choices.
- To avoid a misunderstanding like the one described in the opening scenario, try to have something other than plain cardboard boxes or plastic garbage bags on hand to return bodies in. There are several items that are better alternatives. Blankets or towels, for example, can be bought very inexpensively at yard sales or thrift stores. Inexpensive cardboard caskets and polyethylene body bags made specifically for the veterinary market are also available (see Resources).
- Before clients pick up a pet's cremains, prepare them for what they will see and feel regarding the transformation that has taken place. For many owners, the difference in size, volume, and weight between a furry body and a container of cremains can be shocking and emotionally overwhelming. Encourage the client to bring a friend or family member along and to bring a small box or basket in which to carry the cremains.
- If the client is aware that a pet's death is imminent, as with a scheduled euthanasia, ask him or her to bring something from home in which to

wrap or transport the pet's body. Then you can be certain that the client will feel the item used is appropriate.

- There are times when it may be desirable to perform a necropsy on an animal that has died. Where necropsy is warranted, the option must be tactfully introduced and explained to the client. Several points are relevant to tactful discussions of necropsy:
  - Most pet owners are unfamiliar with the term "necropsy" but are familiar with the term "autopsy" or "postmortem examination." Define the new word in terms of these familiar words.
  - A cosmetic necropsy, in which only selected tissues are removed, is usually recommended when a pet owner wants to find out why the animal died, but also wants the body returned for burial.
  - Whether a necropsy is complete or cosmetic, it should never be performed without an owner's knowledge or permission.

STEP 3 Stay Connected through Follow-up Care

- *Remains retrieval* is a very important and often overlooked aspect of body care following the death of a companion animal. When clients return to the animal hospital to pick up the pet's body or cremated remains, they often have expectations about how this event will be handled, only to experience something completely different. For example, when retrieving remains, some clients want to sit down and talk with one or more of the veterinary professionals who helped them at the time of the death, while others prefer to simply pick up the pet's body or cremains without talking to anyone. Regardless of how clients want the event structured, a warm expression of condolence and support should be provided by whoever delivers the pet's body or cremains to the client.
- If clients wish to schedule an appointment for remains retrieval, it is important to set a time for an office visit. Given the sensitive nature of this meeting, it is probably best not to charge the client for this appointment. When the client arrives, he or she should be taken into a private room—your office, an exam room, or the visitation/euthanasia room—and gently presented with the pet's body or cremains. If possible, use a different room from the one where the client's pet died.
- If you are keeping the animal's body in a cooler until the client can view it or pick it up, curl the body into a sleeplike position so that the

client will be able to place the body in a casket or easily transport it in a car. It's a good idea to keep a box, a vinyl casket, or another container at your clinic for shaping and storage purposes.

- If the client is taking the pet's body home, be sure it is not transported out to the client's car through your busy waiting room.
- It's also important to have the body positioned in a way that is pleasing for clients to see and touch when they say their final goodbye. This usually means placing the body inside a box that is padded with towels or a blanket, a cardboard casket, or an animal body bag and allowing the animal's head to remain outside the container. This preparation also allows clients to quickly and easily enclose the body and to transport it to a car when they are ready to leave your clinic.

ROLE-PLAY IDEAS

For managers and client care specialists: Practice greeting clients who have returned to your clinic to pick up their pet's cremains. Remember to prepare your clients for what they will see and to present the cremains to them.

For veterinary technicians: Practice supporting clients who must make a decision about body care. Describe the different options and normalize their emotions.

For veterinarians: Using a situation similar to the opening scenario, practice talking with clients who are unhappy about some aspect of their pet's body care. Try to find ways to support them and to respond to their anger appropriately. Pay close attention to your verbal and nonverbal communication and to the ways in which you can avoid becoming judgmental or defensive.

Your Notes ✍

SITUATION 8

Client Guilt

Mark McEachern is sitting in an exam room waiting for news about his beagle, Snoopy, who was hit by a car. You knock gently, enter, and explain to him that Snoopy has died. He stares at the wall for a moment, processing the awful news, then looks at you and says, "I knew I should have fixed our gate. It didn't latch right, and Snoopy got out, and now he's dead. . . . I killed him. I'm the one who caused his death. . . . I will never, ever forgive myself."

Assessment: What's Going On Here?

Guilt is the critic, the inner voice that judges one's thoughts, actions, behaviors, decisions, and feelings. Sometimes guilt is justified and other times it is not. Some clients *do* create the circumstances that either directly or indirectly cause their pet's death. For instance, some owners decide to euthanize their pet simply because the pet exhibits unwanted behavior, or because the clients are making a lifestyle change (for example, moving into an apartment). Others may be negligent in the way they care for their pet, or knowingly put their pet in potentially dangerous situations (for example, allowing the pet to ride in the open bed of a pickup truck). When death occurs in these cases, feelings of guilt may be justified.

Other times, guilt is not justified. For example, many clients feel guilty when their pet is diagnosed with a terminal illness. They feel they "should have known" or could have done something to prevent the disease. At the very least, many feel they should have noticed the symptoms sooner. In addition, many clients feel guilty after euthanizing their pet, even if the decision was clearly in the animal's best interests.

In general, guilt usually stems from a client's belief that he or she has breached the contract he or she made with the pet to keep the pet alive, safe, and healthy. The support you offer a client who feels guilty may vary according to whether or not you believe the client's guilt is justified.

Plan

Support Protocol: What to Say, What to Do

STEP 1 Lay the Foundation

- Structure the environment so you and your client can have a private, emotional conversation. During the conversation, use attending behaviors, touch, and paraphrasing, making comments such as, "It sounds as though you had every intention of fixing your gate," and "If I'm hearing you right, Snoopy had never gotten out of your yard before." Listen in an active way to your client.
- Be certain the room is well stocked with tissues as well as client education materials and referral information.

STEP 2 Implement Support Techniques

- Acknowledge the client's feelings of guilt and create opportunities for him or her to talk about them. You cannot change or fix another person's guilty feelings; you can only listen without judgment. For example, in the scenario that opens this situation, instead of saying, "Don't feel so bad," or "It wasn't really your fault," you might say something like "I hear how guilty you feel about Snoopy's death, Mark, and I know you would give anything to be able to go back in time and fix that gate."
- Facilitate a way for the client to say goodbye or even apologize to the pet if the client feels that he or she indirectly caused an accident. You might suggest that the client view the pet's body, go home and write a letter to the pet, or compensate for the negligence by donating to or volunteering for an animal-related organization.
- The guilt that is commonly present when a client decides to euthanize a very sick or injured pet cannot be taken away completely, but it can be minimized. You can gently tell the client that people often use guilt to distract themselves from the more painful feelings of sadness and

loneliness. You can also give the client permission to experience the full range of grief manifestations that accompany loss. Finally, you can remind the client that you consider euthanasia to be a privilege and a gift. For example, "You did everything of a medical nature that you could possibly do for Snoopy and, in the end, you gave him a loving gift—a peaceful, painless death."

- Occasionally, you will see clients who you believe deserve to feel the guilt they are experiencing. Perhaps they have been grossly negligent or even abusive to their pet. In these cases, your goal is not to alleviate the client's guilt, but to act as an advocate for the animal. In most instances, these are not the kinds of clients you want to cultivate. Rather, they are the ones you want to report to the authorities in order to prevent them from owning other animals in the future.

STEP 3 Stay Connected through Follow-up Care

- Even when a client's guilt is not justified, remember that it is not your job (nor is it often even possible) to make guilty feelings go away. No matter what you say, some clients will remain convinced that the little, insignificant things they did or didn't do actually caused their companion animal's death. Clients hang on to these beliefs and their guilt for a multitude of reasons, none of which are within the scope of your ability or responsibility to resolve. The best you can do to support clients who are dealing with unjustified guilt is to patiently and repeatedly review the medical facts pertaining to their pet's death and acknowledge their feelings.
- Most clients who feel guilty also feel embarrassed that they may have harmed their pet by making bad decisions or participating in dangerous activities. Along with their embarrassment, they are probably wondering how their pet's accidental injury or death has affected your opinion of them. If you can separate the person from his or her questionable behavior, you can probably honestly say, for example, "Mr. McEachern, I can see that this mistake is making you feel terribly guilty. But I do believe you are a responsible and conscientious pet owner who never intended to bring any harm to Snoopy. I agree, though, that it's important to keep a secure, safe space for your animal to be in."

- This statement won't do much to alleviate your client's guilt, but it will reassure him that you still support him, won't judge him, and don't wish to see him punish himself over the accident. He will return your kindness and understanding by remaining a loyal client—and, one would hope, by fixing the latch on his gate!

ROLE-PLAY IDEAS

For hospital managers and client care specialists: Using the opening case scenario, try talking to the fictional Mr. McEachern about his feelings of guilt over Snoopy's death. Practice ways you can acknowledge his feelings without telling him outright not to feel guilty.

For veterinary technicians: Practice talking with Mr. McEachern about his guilt and how he blames himself for Snoopy's death. Then practice talking with a client who feels guilty about waiting too long before making the decision for euthanasia.

For veterinarians: Practice talking with clients who feel guilty for a variety of reasons. For accidental deaths you can use the opening scenario to practice helping Mr. McEachern deal with his feelings about Snoopy's death. Additionally, practice talking with a client who feels guilty about his or her pet's death due to a sudden illness, such as cancer. You can also practice talking with a client who feels guilty about the euthanasia (such as waiting too long or euthanizing too early).

Your Notes ✍

SITUATION 9

Making Referrals

Joan, a good client of many years, doesn't seem to be handling the loss of her cat very well. When you ask her about it, she replies, "My daughter died three years ago and Betsy was her cat. That cat slept on the bed beside my daughter every day while she was sick. Losing Betsy is like losing Janie all over again. . . . I don't think I can bear to feel the grief again."

Assessment: What's Going On Here?

In the opening scenario, the cat's death represents what is called a *symbolic loss*. A symbolic loss is one that is associated with a previous loss in life. A companion animal may represent a pet owner's last living link to a special person, place, thing, or time in life. The pet's death can destroy that living link.

Although pet loss is significant in its own right, the grief the client feels may be greater when the loss triggers memories of a previous loss than when no previous loss is associated with the pet. Symbolic losses are just one of many types of loss that can complicate the grieving process. A variety of factors may be present when a pet dies that intensify the grieving process, make the grieving last longer than usual, and/or cause it to be reactivated more easily later than when no complicating factors exist. Clients who experience pet loss that is symbolic, traumatic, unexpected, or complicated in some way by its association with other difficult circumstances are good candidates for referral to mental health professionals and grief support programs.

Plan

Support Protocol: What to Say, What to Do

STEP 1 Lay the Foundation

- Assess which of your clients may be in need of extended support via referral by examining factors present in the client's history and current circumstances. These factors may include:
    - The strength of the client's bond with the pet
    - The circumstances surrounding the pet's death
    - The client's personal loss history and support system
    - The client's ability to cope
    - When one or more of these factors seem to be suspect, the client is probably a good candidate for referral. For example, if you have had previous conversations with a client about her child who recently died and the solace she found in the company of her dog, your assessment of her need for further support would probably be high.
- Screen your referral resources prior to your need for them. Not all mental health professionals understand or are skilled in working with issues of grief. Likewise, not all grief counselors are sympathetic to issues of pet loss and pet owner grief. If you are interested in teaming up with a mental health professional, it is important to get to know something about your potential candidates and to choose wisely.
- There are many ways to make professional support available to clients. However, even if professional support exists, it won't be of help if you are uncomfortable making referrals. Practice stock phrases you can use to let clients know about the human service resources that are available. Be sure to pair these words with nonverbal helping techniques such as touch, direct eye contact, and other attending behaviors.

STEP 2 Implement Support Techniques

- In cases like the one in the opening scenario, it is not your responsibility to meet your clients' needs for ongoing grief education and support. These kinds of cases go beyond what you are qualified to do. This is a good time to refer clients to a professional grief therapist or grief support group. One of the most effective ways to do this is to give every client who experiences pet loss a packet of written materials describing local support groups, pet-loss counselors, and pet-loss support hotlines. With referral names, addresses, and telephone numbers in hand, clients are made aware of the resources available to them and can choose for themselves which, if any, of these services would benefit them.

- Another way you can make referrals is on a case-by-case basis. When speaking directly to a client who could benefit from further support, you can use self-disclosure and say something like "I know how hard Betsy's death is for you. I work with a person who specializes in helping pet owners deal with the grief they feel after their pet dies, especially in a situation like yours where there is a connection between Betsy and Janie. Many of my clients talk with her at least once, and it seems to help a great deal. I talk with her about cases that are tough for me, too. I'd like to give you her name and number."
- Normalize your client's grief by saying something like "It sounds as though the connection between Janie's death and Betsy's death is complicating your grief. This is actually very common. I know your feelings can be sorted out, but I'm just not trained in this area. I do know someone who can help you, though. I know her well and recommend her highly. Shall we call her now to see if she has some time free, or would you like me to have her call you?"
- Many adults will seek help for their children or for another member of their family even if they are reluctant to ask for help for themselves. You might say something like "Joan, I know you and Paul have other children. Have you thought about how you might help them cope with the connection between Janie's and Betsy's deaths? There are some really effective ways to help children deal with loss, and I work with a woman who can provide you with this information. Here's her name and number." This is called the "back-door" approach and is usually less threatening for clients, since they do not perceive the referral as aimed directly at them.

Suicide Ideation versus Suicide Intent

Although thoughts and comments about suicide are quite common, truly suicidal clients are very rare. Sometimes clients will say something like the following: "Life means nothing to me without Pepper. Sometimes I wonder why I should go on . . ." A remark like that is usually a normal reaction to loss. These comments are called suicide ideation and are simply an indication of the griever's deep feelings of despair. Many pet owners draw companionship and emotional comfort from their pet and it is difficult for them to imagine what their daily routine will be like without their pet. Losing such significant relationships can feel overwhelming.

On rare occasions, there may be suicidal intent underlying a client's comments about wanting to die. This means that a client may be seriously considering suicide. If you are concerned that a client has a suicidal intent, you may ask him or her. For example: "Joan, you've told me how devastated you are feeling right now, and I'm concerned about you. Do you really feel like you might harm yourself right now?" It's important for you to know how to determine the difference between a normal grief reaction (suicide ideation) and a grief response that is abnormal or extreme (suicidal intent). You also need to know how to help in the latter situation.

Most people who attempt suicide are ambivalent about the act. They don't really want to kill themselves; they just want to find an end to their overwhelming feelings of pain and distress. A common myth about intervening with suicidal people is that if you ask people directly about their suicidal comments, you'll somehow condone the act and encourage them to kill themselves. Yet, the opposite is actually true. Open, honest discussions about suicide can lower people's anxiety level; help them feel they are understood, cared about, and supported; and make the event less likely to occur.

To attend to clients who verbalize suicidal intent, you need to find the courage to ask specific questions about how they feel and why they would want to die. During this conversation, you shouldn't use euphemisms like "pass away" or "cross over." Euphemisms indicate that you feel anxious talking about the subject matter at hand. If you are too anxious to talk about suicide, you won't be able to help your client deal realistically with these feelings.

As with other situations in which you need to communicate with grieving clients, you'll want to lay a foundation. Occasionally, a client who is preparing for suicide may bring one or more of his or her pets in for euthanasia so the pets will not be left without care. If a healthy animal is scheduled for euthanasia, it's very important to ask why your client is requesting that the animal be killed. Before you begin this conversation, it's a good idea to structure your environment by asking your client to join you in a private, comfortable room where you are better able to talk and assess the situation. Treat this conversation as you would treat an emergency. Alert your staff to your change in schedule and, since pets can be a distraction, ask a staff member to remove the pet while you speak with the client.

Next, you'll want to implement support techniques. Acknowledge every comment containing suicide ideation and take it seriously. Paraphrase what your client has just said, perhaps by saying, "It sounds like you can't imagine life without Pepper." Be direct and push yourself to ask the tough questions. Too many questions can make you sound nervous or like an interrogator. Simply say, "Mary, some of the comments you're making concern me. Are you thinking of taking your own life now that Pepper has died?" Most often your client will say (perhaps with some embarrassment or anger), "No, of course not. I'm just so upset—I didn't want to lose him." In this case, you can relax and be quite sure that your client's comments represent a normal grief reaction. You might say, "I'm glad to hear that. We take these comments very seriously here, and I always feel it is my responsibility to ask people what they mean when they make them."

However, if the answer is "Yes, I've thought about it occasionally. She's all I have," you will need to facilitate an intervention and/or referral by taking the following steps:

1. Assess the lethality of your client's situation (see textbox "Assessing Suicidal Lethality").
2. Support your client through the immediate crisis.
3. Refer your client to an appropriate mental health professional or social service agency or contact the appropriate crisis intervention resource yourself.

If you believe that your client is not in immediate danger, ask him or her to call a crisis or suicide hotline, a friend or relative, a family physician, a member of the clergy, or a therapist while in your presence. If the client declines to reach out, you may choose to call one of these individuals yourself on his or her behalf. If you decide you must notify someone, always tell your client. Explain that if he or she is unwilling to make the call, you will make the call. If you say this in a firm, supportive way rather than in a scolding or threatening manner, most clients will agree to your offer of help or decide to call someone themselves.

The best strategy to use if you encounter a truly suicidal client is to get help immediately. In most communities, professional help is not hard to find. There are suicide or crisis intervention centers staffed with well-trained people who can provide you with advice or debriefing. In addition, most mental health agencies have a professional on staff who is authorized to hospitalize people on a short-term basis for observation and for their own protection. Many hospitals offer this service, too.

The most effective and immediate help you can get is the police. The rule of thumb regarding whether or not to contact law enforcement authorities is to do so whenever someone makes a serious threat to do harm to self or others. This is the code most police officers use as a guide for intervening in potentially dangerous situations. When they learn that you are concerned about a potential suicide, the police may do what is called a welfare check. This means they will locate your client and either intervene to prevent a suicide that is taking place or interview your client further to make sure the danger of suicide is not imminent.

continues

Suicide Ideation versus Suicide Intent, continued

How aggressive you should be in connecting a potentially suicidal client with appropriate help depends in part on what is called the lethality of the situation (see textbox "Assessing Suicidal Lethality").

When providing client support, some people attempt to make a contract with a suicidal client, insisting that a client agree to call them before carrying through with a suicide plan. This is not a good idea for veterinary professionals. If a client calls you when the lethality of the situation is high, you may quickly be in over your head in terms of your training and capabilities. In addition, if you receive a call from a suicidal client, you may also be tempted to go to him or her in order to try to prevent the suicide. However, you should never go to a client's house or attempt to rescue the client, no matter where he or she may be. There is always the potential for suicidal clients to turn homicidal, and your own life could be in danger if you attempt any kind of direct help.

The odds are high that you will never encounter a truly suicidal client. If you do, you should talk with a trained mental health or social service professional who can advise you about what actions to take and about who can also support you. Being involved in someone's attempted or completed suicide can be emotionally devastating for you. If it happens, you need to take care of yourself and talk to someone about it. No one can assume responsibility for someone else's life. You will need to be reassured that you were not responsible, either directly or indirectly, for your client's decision to end his or her life.

STEP 3 Stay Connected through Follow-up Care

- You may need to refer a client to a mental health professional, social worker, or pet-loss support group several times before he or she is ready to actually talk with one. For many people, there is a stigma attached to talking to a counselor. Thus, they avoid the encounter for as long as possible. However, clients who are reluctant to seek professional help are often the ones who continue to ask you to help them with their grief. It's important for you to continue to abide by the principles of your paraprofessional helping role. This means you need to sensitively, but consistently, decline to provide these clients with further help and continue to refer them to the counselor with whom you work, regardless of whether or not they actually seek help.

Assessing Suicidal Lethality

1. Determine whether or not your client has a specific plan and how quickly he or she could put a plan into action. For instance, has your client collected medication and determined the dosage that would be fatal? Does your client now have the bottle of pills in hand, or would the client need to first obtain a prescription and then go to the drugstore to pick up the medication?
2. Assess whether or not the method your client has chosen has a high probability of quick success. For example, is your client planning to take pills that would be relatively slow-acting, or does he or she plan to use a handgun that is already loaded with ammunition?
3. Ascertain whether or not your client is isolated and alone or lives in close proximity to someone who can help.
4. If the danger level for your client (or others) is high, call the police and other professionals who can be of immediate help to you and your client. If you are talking to your client on the telephone, try to stay on the call while another staff member alerts the police and other appropriate resources.

ROLE-PLAY IDEAS

For hospital managers and client care specialists: Use the opening scenario to practice supporting a client by referring her to outside support. Be sure to normalize and acknowledge the client's feelings.

For veterinary technicians: Use the opening scenario to practice how you would tie Betsy's and Janie's deaths together and encourage the client to contact a counselor or grief support group. Also practice supporting a client who feels overwhelmed by sadness and expresses *suicide ideation* (thoughts and feelings of despair and "endings"). Be sure to ask the tough questions about the client's intentions and make a referral or help the client find outside help. Alert your veterinarian to this conversation and bring him or her up-to-date regarding the client's comments and your referrals.

continues

ROLE-PLAY IDEAS, continued

For veterinarians: Use the opening scenario to practice normalizing the client's grief over Betsy and Janie. Provide good grief education and practice phrases or methods you can rely on for making referrals. For example, most clients are familiar with the process of being referred to an ancillary health care service in human medicine. You might say something like "Joan, if you had a broken arm, you wouldn't walk around for three weeks without having it looked at. The same is true with a broken heart. I know someone who can help you with the process of healing from both Janie's death and Betsy's death. Let's call her now and see if she can set up an appointment to see you today or tomorrow."

Practice talking with a client who expresses suicidal intent. Assess for lethality and then practice supporting the client based on this information. Try making a referral, calling a resource to get your client outside help, and calling the police to get immediate help.

Your Notes

SITUATION 10

Helping Children

Your client Mrs. Smith is trying to calm down her young son, Jimmy, after the death of their cat, Midas. Standing over him, she murmurs, "Jimmy, the doctor couldn't save Midas. He was too badly hurt when the car hit him, and he's gone now. We can't see him anymore." But Jimmy cries, "No, no! I don't believe you! Midas is in that room! I want to see him!" Then Jimmy collapses onto the floor, crying, kicking, and flailing his arms.

Mrs. Smith, still standing, explains, "You can't see him, Jimmy. Midas is gone." "He is not gone!" Jimmy screams. "You're lying! I want my Midas!"

Assessment: What's Going On Here?

Children often grieve just as deeply as adults. However, until children reach the age of eight or nine, most do not possess the ability to think rationally about death or to verbally express their needs and feelings surrounding their grief. Thus, many children act out their grief through pretending, drawing pictures or telling stories, or even misbehaving. Expressions of anger and irritability, such as Jimmy's tantrum in the example above, are often due to the child's feelings of confusion and loss of control and his or her inability to verbally express these feelings.

Cases involving children are tricky. Some parents view any suggestion about how to help their children through the grief process as unwanted interference. Your well-meaning comments about how to deal with children's grief may put some parents on the defensive, especially if they think you are criticizing their values or parenting styles.

However, most parents sincerely want to help their children and will be open to your ideas if you offer them in a gentle way. This is a good time to acknowledge whatever a client is already doing to include a child in the grieving process and to normalize the child's behaviors and feelings. This acknowledgment lets parents know you recognize that they want to be responsible, protective parents. If you have children yourself, you can also use a brief self-disclosure story, relating any methods you have used to help your own children deal with pet loss.

Plan
Support Protocol: What to Say, What to Do

STEP 1 Lay the Foundation

- Educate parents about children and grief *before* their pets die. Remember, most people operate from a host of misconceptions about normal grief. When parents are uninformed about normal grief and the best ways to prepare children to deal with it, they may expect too much from their children (or leave them out entirely) and inadvertently cause them emotional harm.
- If you are not comfortable educating parents about the needs of children before pet loss occurs, refer them to a reputable website or local grief counselor who has experience helping others to face pet loss. You can also make books and videotapes about helping children deal with pet loss available to your clients. (See the Resources section at the back of this book.)
- Encourage parents to include children in decision-making and to trust and honor their children's requests. With preparation and support, even young children benefit from making their own decisions and facing their own fears. If a child wishes to attend the euthanasia of his or her pet or to view the pet's body after it dies, it is usually better to allow this than not to. As long as the child is well prepared for what he or she will see and do at these times, and supported emotionally throughout each experience, these are ways of helping the child to say goodbye to a beloved pet.

- Encourage parents to be honest with their children. When parents lie to their children about a pet's death, it is not because they are malicious, but because they want to protect their children from further pain. The lie, in their minds, serves to blunt the harsh reality that would frighten the child. Yet, lies create confusion and mistrust. If parents ask *you* to collude with them in a lie about a pet's medical condition or death, please interpret the request as a plea for help. Gently decline to do so and use gentle confrontation, immediacy, and written materials to offer to assist parents in telling their children the truth about the pet.

STEP 2 Implement Support Techniques

- If, like the scenario at the beginning of this section, the situation requires immediate intervention, use touch, direct eye contact, and attending behaviors to calm the child and active listening to really hear what the child is asking for. Then, as much as possible, advocate for the child's needs to be met. Before you intervene, remind yourself to be kind, respectful, and nonjudgmental. Don't take sides, and be sure your voice does not have a scolding tone.
  - For example, in the opening scenario, you might use touch and eye contact to gain both the parent's and Jimmy's attention. You could squat down to be at Jimmy's eye level and then, speaking slowly and softly, say, "Jimmy, Mrs. Smith, I can see how sad and difficult this is for both of you." Then, structure the environment by getting them to somewhere more private. If necessary, take Jimmy's hand. Guide the parent by placing your hand on her arm or even putting your arm around her shoulders as you lead them toward a private area. You might say, "I'd like you both to come with me to a room where we can talk about Midas and decide what we can do to help you say goodbye to him. Jimmy, I promise we won't move Midas until we've all decided what to do." Once settled, you can facilitate a consensus regarding how everyone involved can best have their needs met.
- If a companion animal has been injured and is cut, bloody, or disfigured in some way, take time to clean the blood away, bandage a wound, or at least remove the medical equipment you were using to try to save the animal's life. Then, after explaining to the parent that it

is often beneficial for children to view a pet's body, and with parental permission, prepare the child with a description of the wounds and/or physical changes he or she is likely to see and offer the opportunity to say a last goodbye. Even though the pet has already died, viewing their pet's body is almost always helpful to children because it helps them accept the reality of the pet's death.

- When speaking with children, avoid using euphemisms and clichés like "put to sleep" and "gone to heaven." Young children take what adults say literally. If they think their pet is sleeping, they also think it will soon wake up. In addition, for young children who go to sleep every night, associating going to sleep with never waking up can be a scary thought.
- During euthanasia, young children may cry one minute and ask if they can play outdoors the next. Suggest that parents ask a family friend or child-care provider to accompany them to your clinic the day of their pet's euthanasia. This way, young children can be cared for while parents complete their goodbyes with their pets.

STEP 3 Stay Connected through Follow-up Care

- Being an instrumental part of teaching children how to face death and grief is the epitome of providing client support. There is simply nothing more satisfying. If you're successful, you'll help parents create more emotionally healthy children and more positive experiences with veterinary medicine.
- Direct your written condolences to the children as well as the parents. Children often hold veterinary professionals responsible for their pet's death. When this happens, they can influence their parents' choice of veterinarian by resisting any future interactions with you. When you support your young clients, they remain loyal and grateful to you and your staff.
- If you provide special keepsakes or memorials like clay pawprints, consider making one for each child in addition to the one you make for the family.
- If parents ask your advice about adopting a new pet, it's helpful to remind them that most children (and adults!) need time to grieve for their pet who has died and do not always want to immediately adopt

another one. Presenting children with new pets too soon gives them the impression that loved ones who die are not unique or special and are easily replaced.

Understanding Grief and Children

The experience of pet loss during childhood is not a "dress rehearsal" for learning how to deal with "more important" losses later on. Pet loss can be just as significant as the loss of a human family member, so it should be acknowledged and not trivialized.

Infants (birth to 1 year)

Babies probably do not respond to grief because they have not yet reached a stage of cognitive development that would allow them to understand that a loss has occurred. Babies do, however, react to increased tension in the home and will commonly express it by crying, withdrawing, clinging, or even regressing developmentally. During times of family grieving, the best support for babies is reassurance, cuddling, and maintaining their usual routines as much as possible.

Toddlers and Preschoolers (2 to 4 years)

Young children do not understand the permanence of death, so they often ask when their pet is coming back. Toddlers are curious and relaxed about death and ask lots of questions. While young children probably don't really grieve, they do react to the grief of others around them. These reactions are often expressed through misbehavior, an increased need for attention, and imaginary play (such as pretending to bury a pet). If young children are discouraged or prevented from finding an outlet for their grief, they may develop psychosomatic complaints (for example, stomachaches).

Like babies, toddlers need to be reassured and kept to their routines as much as possible. They also benefit from honest conversations about their pet and activities like drawing pictures of their pet as ways to express their grief.

School-Aged Children (5 to 12 years)

At these ages, children are usually conditioned to the prevailing cultural and familial views and taboos that surround death. Some fear death. Others taunt it, believing they can hide, run away, or control death the way superheroes do on TV. Around the age of 8, kids gain a cognitive understanding of death and realize it is both permanent and universal. With this realization, young children grieve just as intensely as adults, but they may do so more sporadically because of their shorter attention span.

School-aged children are helped when adults involve them in their pet's treatments and in the decisions surrounding euthanasia and saying goodbye. They are also helped when adults provide opportunities for them to talk and to ask questions

continues

Understanding Grief and Children, continued

about death, as well as when seeing adults openly and honestly express their feelings of grief.

Adolescents (13 to 17 years)

Teens are unpredictable, self-conscious, and prone to mood swings. Their grief responses are often confusing and contradictory. Adolescents need opportunities to express their grief verbally. If they do not have a chance to discuss their feelings, their grief can be complicated by unresolved feelings of guilt and anger. Like younger children, they can also develop psychosomatic complaints. Adults should create opportunities for teens to talk about their grief and allow them to participate actively in decisions about end-of-life care for the pet as well as after-death arrangements such as viewing the body or planning a memorial.

Young Adults (18 to 21 years)

Young adults are often overlooked in terms of their need for adult assistance following the death of a pet. Yet, the impact on them is often great and they are still young enough to need special attention. For many young adults, the death of a childhood pet is a rite of passage—the passage of their own childhood. They may feel guilty for "abandoning" their companion animal when they left home and resentful if they were not told about its decline in health or included in decisions regarding treatment and/or euthanasia. Like adolescents, young adults benefit from open, honest discussions; active and equal participation; and opportunities to say goodbye to their friend.

ROLE-PLAY IDEAS

For hospital managers and client care specialists: Use the opening scenario to practice supporting Mrs. Smith and Jimmy. Normalize and acknowledge feelings and practice using child-friendly language.

For veterinary technicians: Use the opening scenario to practice how you would support Mrs. Smith and Jimmy. Practice how you might refer Mrs. Smith to a counselor or grief support. Practice talking with Jimmy about Midas and see what his level of understanding is about death. Practice offering support.

For veterinarians: Use the opening scenario to help Mrs. Smith and normalize Jimmy's grief reaction about Midas to both of them. Provide helpful grief education and practice phrases or methods you can rely on for making referrals.

Practice talking with Mrs. Smith about Jimmy's level of understanding of death and grief. Answer sample questions a parent might ask in this situation.

Your Notes

SITUATION 11

Helping Seniors

Mrs. Franklin is an elderly woman who lives alone and has been a client of yours for many years. Her beloved dog, Toby, whom she refers to as her "one and only companion," is dying from kidney disease. You talk with Mrs. Franklin and she decides to euthanize Toby. She tells you that once Toby is gone, she'll be "completely alone." You gently touch her arm and say, "I can see that this is going to be a difficult time for you, Mrs. Franklin." She nods and then adds, "I don't have anyone to help me with Toby's body. Would you consider coming to my house and burying him for me?"

Assessment: What's Going On Here?

Mrs. Franklin is facing a difficult predicament, but it is not an unusual one. Like many senior citizens, she lacks physical strength, has a minimal support system, and does not know where to turn for help. Naturally, she turns to the veterinary team member who has been most involved in her pet's care.

As people age, their physical strength and stamina decline, making them incapable of undertaking all the activities they did in their younger days. Memory losses due to aging or disease can also occur. Retirement may bring a change in standard of living. Older people living on fixed incomes may not be able to afford treatment for their pets and may be forced to make life-and-death decisions based on finances. They may also have lost the majority of their emotional support network. Spouses and friends may have died, and children and other relatives may live far away. As a result, older people may need extra support, time, care, and understanding when their pet is ill or has died.

To help them fill in the gaps, you can keep a reference list of resources in your community for senior citizens. This could include transportation services, drugstores and pet shops that offer senior discounts, and social service agencies or volunteers who are willing to assist seniors with unexpected needs like burying a cat or dog.

Plan

Support Protocol: What to Say, What to Do

STEP 1 Lay the Foundation

- Structure the environment so older clients can be safe and comfortable during their pet's appointments. Examples include altering seating arrangements for greater comfort and adapting walkways to make it easier to move in and out of the exam room. Have tissues and water on hand, and try to minimize noise as much as possible so clients can focus with fewer distractions.
- Be aware that elderly pet owners may have had numerous experiences with pet death, companion-animal euthanasia, and viewing bodies over the years. Unfortunately, those situations may have been poorly handled, leaving elderly owners skeptical about your offers to provide grief support. In these cases, their current decisions (not to be present at euthanasia, not to view their pet's body) may be based on outdated information and previous negative experiences. With gentle persistence and education, you may be able to give them a new, much more positive experience with pet loss.
- Respect the years of learning that elderly people have, and remember that they are all individuals with their own levels of education, life experiences, and mental and physical competencies. Don't assume older clients need special consideration until you have asked them directly or observed a decline in their functioning for yourself. Remember, too, that because of generational differences and the social climate in which they were raised, elderly pet owners may have more discomfort with the open expression of emotion than do younger clients.

- Encourage elderly clients to consider enriching their lives by having more than one pet if they are so inclined and able to care for them. This can provide additional happiness, relief from loneliness, and critical support after one of the pets in the home has died.

STEP 2 Implement Support Strategies

- If you have laid the groundwork and have a list of volunteers who can help seniors with special tasks, you can assure someone like Mrs. Franklin that people will be available to help her. You could say, for example, "Don't you worry, Mrs. Franklin. I know of a lovely service club whose members have volunteered to help with things like this. I'm sure they will be willing to come and help you bury Toby when the time comes, if that is what you would like to do." Then, you can tell her about other body-care options, such as cremation. You can also ask her more about what things will be like when the beloved pet is gone, using your support skills to help prepare her for this change in her lifestyle.
- Repeat information several times, if necessary, since older clients may be hard of hearing or may need extra time to understand what is being said. It may also be helpful for you to write out information or instructions, as elderly people may not be able to remember detailed information once they leave your clinic. Older persons living alone may want to call a relative or friend to help them make a decision about the pet's care.
- Older clients may reminisce about the past and engage you in conversations more than do people in other age groups. They may tell you about other pets or family members who have died. Discussions may also include comments about their own health or the acknowledgment that their own life is drawing to a close. If you can, schedule a bit more time for these appointments and don't trivialize the importance of these conversations. Older people are often lonely and benefit from honest, open conversations with another human being. Discussions about death can also be helpful, when they arise, and may provide older people with an important but rare opportunity to tell someone how they feel about aging and dying. Although thinking

about death may sound morose to younger people, these conversations are actually comforting and helpful to older people. When clients say something like "I suppose I'll be dying soon, too," a response like "Oh, Mrs. Franklin, you'll live forever" is not helpful. Instead of brushing off the comment or changing the subject, try saying something like "Well, Mrs. Franklin, when you do die—and I hope it's not for a very long time—I will miss you."

- For older pet owners, companion animals are often symbolically linked with deceased loved ones. Perhaps the dog now dying was an anniversary present from a spouse who has died, or the elderly cat may have belonged to a deceased sibling. Many older people have not fully grieved all of their losses. Thus, when an older person is faced with the death of a companion animal, it is likely that some unresolved grief will be triggered, as well as fears and anxieties about the person's own death. Keep your referral list handy and help older clients find resources that are appropriate for them.

STEP 3 Stay Connected through Follow-up Care

- Companion animals have a positive effect on the physical and emotional well-being of older people. In fact, relationships between pets and the elderly have been shown to be so beneficial that laws have changed nationally to allow elderly pet owners to keep pets in retirement centers, nursing homes, and federally funded public housing. If pets provide significant health benefits for older people, the deaths of pets most likely affect their health as well. Check in with your older clients as often as you can after they've lost a pet.
- Although replacing a pet is not an effective remedy for grief, there are so many benefits of pet ownership for seniors that, in this case, it may be a good idea. If it is appropriate for your older client to adopt another pet, you might recommend a specific breed that you think would fit the individual's abilities and lifestyle.

ROLE-PLAY IDEAS

For hospital managers and client care specialists: Using the above scenario, practice talking with Mrs. Franklin about Toby's illness and what things will be like for her when Toby dies. Practice your support skills while still maintaining your professional boundaries.

For veterinary technicians: Practice how you would support Mrs. Franklin and answer questions that she may have about Toby or the euthanasia. Make appropriate referrals.

For veterinarians: Using the above scenario, practice supporting your client and answering her question about burying her dog for her. Use your verbal and nonverbal communication to support her while preserving your professional boundaries. Practice making referrals for support.

Your Notes

SITUATION 12

Helping Disabled Clients

Mr. Cooper is a long-standing client who has Parkinson's disease and uses a wheelchair. His companion and assistance dog, Clyde, is dying from cancer, and all treatment options have been exhausted. Mr. Cooper brings Clyde to you for euthanasia because he feels that it's the best way to keep Clyde from suffering. Mr. Cooper tells you that he's worried about how he will manage life without Clyde's daily help and companionship. He asks you for advice on what to do.

Assessment: What's Going On Here?

Treating and euthanizing service animals for people with disabilities require extra consideration from the entire veterinary practice team. If clients are visually or hearing-impaired, or have other disabilities, their pet and/or service animal can be incredibly important in their lives. Not only do service animals provide companionship, they also give their owners a level of independence and functioning that would be difficult to achieve without them. Because of the work these animals do and the impact they have on their owners' lives, it's not unusual for some people with disabilities to view their pets almost as extensions of themselves. Therefore, the death of a service animal may result in a loss of self-confidence, self-esteem, and freedom, along with all the other common responses to grief.

Mr. Cooper in the above example probably has a number of concerns when he asks for advice. Most people in his situation would be experiencing anticipatory grief. Someone who uses a service animal would also be wondering how to go about finding another animal who will be as loyal and well trained as the one that is dying, and would be wondering how to cope during the transition period. Getting another dog in these cases is a necessity, not just an option to be pondered, and it is a matter that must be dealt with as soon as possible.

Plan
Support Protocol: What to Do, What to Say

STEP 1 Lay the Foundation

- When making treatment decisions about service animals, consider the way in which a particular drug, surgery, or other procedure will affect the animal's ability to work. For instance, a service dog's condition may be treatable, but the treatment may not allow the dog to continue as a service animal. Also, when treatment fails and euthanasia is imminent, people with disabilities may be very sensitive to the way you talk about the animal's quality-of-life issues. It's very important not to give the message that a life with physical impairments is not worth living.
- When a service animal dies, people with disabilities usually can't wait until they are emotionally ready to adopt another pet. Your client may need a new service animal immediately if he or she is to remain independent and continue to engage in daily routines. Owners might have difficulty in bonding with the new animal, however, because they must grieve the deceased animal at the same time they are getting used to and training the new one. These clients can benefit from extra grief support regarding the companion that has died.
- Consider the following in assisting disabled clients:
    - Be sure that your veterinary hospital is accessible. This includes your entrance, examination rooms, restrooms, and other client areas.
    - Be flexible when scheduling appointments. Many disabled people cannot drive and rely on public transportation or rides from friends. They may not be able to meet a tight schedule.

  - Structure your environment carefully to meet the specific needs of disabled clients. A hearing-impaired person, for example, might need a pad of paper or a pencil if he or she does not have an interpreter.
  - Consider assigning a staff member to assist the client with his or her individual needs throughout the entire appointment.

STEP 2 Implement Support Techniques

- Suggest that clients contact appropriate service animal organizations (such as the Delta Society) to help them before their current service animal becomes unable to work because of illness, old age, or death. These organizations can help with locating new animals as well as with the unique grief of dealing with the death of a beloved service companion (and everyday companion!).
- Encourage clients to share their fears, concerns, and feelings with you, and let them know you won't judge them about those emotions. The death or impending death of a service animal is a complex issue with special considerations.

STEP 3 Stay Connected through Follow-up Care

- After a euthanasia, follow up with your client right away. Take a bit of extra time to provide condolences, grief support, and support for any additional issues.
- At some point you may want to inquire if the client has gotten a new service animal, and if so, how things are going with that transition. Be sure to let the client know that you still care and want to help even after a death. Be open to his or her questions or concerns, and make referrals, when appropriate.
- If you talk with the client about a new service animal, this might be a good time to encourage him or her to bring the new animal in for a medical checkup. This type of appointment will give you more time to see how the client is making the transition and determine whether he or she has any concerns about bonding with the new animal.

Communicating with Disabled Clients

There are several factors to consider in communicating with disabled clients. Following are strategies you might try.

For the physically impaired:

- Speak directly to the client rather than to a helper or interpreter.
- Do not assume that a person with a disability always needs assistance in moving around. You can offer help, then let the client decide for him- or herself whether to accept it.
- Ask or wait to be instructed as to how you can help if assistance is requested.
- Never treat people with disabilities as though they were children, and never talk about them as though they were not in the room.
- Use everyday language and don't make a big deal about a slip-up if you inadvertently refer to a person's specific disability (such as saying, "I've gotta run" when speaking with a client who uses a wheelchair).
- When talking with a client in a wheelchair, sit down to place yourself at eye level. Understand that people in wheelchairs often see their chairs as extensions of themselves. Never try to touch, lean on, or hang on to it when talking with them.
- People in wheelchairs may not be able to see what is happening to their companion on an examination table that is higher than they are. If possible, lower the table or tell the client what you are doing.

For the hearing-impaired:

- Get the attention of a person who is hearing-impaired by tapping him or her lightly on the shoulder or waving your hand.
- When speaking, look directly at the client and speak clearly. If a client is able to read lips, keep your hands and other objects away from your face when speaking and stand or sit where you are easily visible.
- Write down important items that you want the client to remember, such as the pet's diagnosis, treatment plan options, and cost estimates.
- When doing a client-present euthanasia, you might want to designate a touch on the arm or other signal to indicate when you will be injecting the drugs. This allows the person to focus on the pet without having to watch you.

For the visually impaired:

- As you enter a room with a client who is blind, identify yourself and anyone else who may be with you.
- Use a normal speaking voice. Most visually impaired people can hear as well as you do, so there is no need to raise your voice.
- During client-present euthanasia, be sure to verbally describe each step, let the client know when you are about to inject the drug, and pronounce the animal dead out loud.

ROLE-PLAY IDEAS

For hospital managers and client care specialists: Role-play the situation in the opening scenario and practice helping a client with a specific disability. Monitor your verbal and nonverbal skills and practice what you might say. Notice whether there are awkward moments that you could learn to deal with more constructively. Consider the different needs of visually impaired clients versus hearing-impaired clients.

For veterinary technicians: Practice talking to a disabled client about euthanasia, and then role-play a situation in which the client is upset or distraught. Practice talking about euthanasia and adopting a new service animal with a client who has a physical disability.

For veterinarians: Practice responding to the situation described above, paying close attention to your verbal and nonverbal communication. Practice supporting a disabled client who has just lost a service dog, paying close attention to how you respond to that person's grief as well as to the disruption in his or her lifestyle.

Your Notes

SITUATION 13

Other Pets' Grief

It's Mr. Taylor's first visit to your clinic since Mack, his golden retriever, died. Today, he's here for a wellness check for Nellie, his black lab. He says, "You know, Nellie has been acting strange ever since Mack died. She won't eat or drink unless I stand right next to her, and she's torn up the carpet in every entryway of our house. Is it possible she's upset about Mack being gone?"

Assessment: What's Going On Here?

Animals in the same household often develop strong bonds with one another and, when separated, can exhibit stress reactions like the ones described above. The grief responses of companion animals have not been scientifically studied, but dozens of anecdotes describing similar behaviors of surviving pets have been reported. Some of the hallmark characteristics commonly thought of as "grief" in companion animals are listed here:

- Anxiety, restlessness, or a need to stay close to the owner
- Changes in eating, drinking, sleeping, or exercise habits
- Signs of depression, such as heavy sighing or lack of interest in usual activities
- Destructive behaviors
- High-pitched distress vocalizations (especially in young animals)
- House soiling
- Searching the yard, house, and other familiar areas for the animal that has died

Many of the "grief" expressions displayed by companion animals seem similar to those of human grief. However, there can also be a complete absence of symptoms in a pet following another pet's death. For this reason and others, "grief" displayed by animals cannot exactly be equated to human grief.

Some clients want to let their surviving pets see and even smell the body of a pet who has died. In fact, some even want to bring their surviving pets to their dying animal's euthanasia. Although there is no scientific evidence that this has any effect on surviving animals, it is sometimes helpful to clients. If your clients feel strongly about involving their pets in this way, why not encourage them to do so? Agreeing to accommodate requests like this can help clients trust you to provide the kind of grief support that is exactly right for them.

Plan

Support Protocol: What to Do, What to Say

STEP 1 Lay the Foundation

- Acknowledge that it is possible for animals to grieve for one another, and validate your client's concern for his or her surviving pet. You might say, "I think it's very possible that Nellie misses Mack. I'm sure it's difficult for you to see Nellie so lonely and upset all the time."
- Normalize your client's concerns. Use self-disclosure if you've experienced a similar situation by saying, for example, "You know, many of our clients tell us about situations similar to yours. When my pet Celia died, my other pet, Millie, went through the same kind of adjustment you're describing." Some clients feel foolish when they assign human characteristics to their animals. Therefore, they are likely to find your nonjudgmental validation of their observations very supportive.
- Educate clients about what may happen in the household if there are two or more surviving pets—for example, a new "alpha" may be established and the "pecking order" of the household may change as the remaining pets adjust to the death of their former companion.

STEP 2 Implement Support Techniques

- Educate clients about normal animal behaviors, such as pack behavior and separation anxiety. Based on what is known about separation reactions and animal behavior, some logical assumptions about modifying or minimizing an animal's negative behaviors can be made. You might suggest that clients try the following:

- Keep the surviving pets' daily routines the same. Animals usually respond well to environments that are predictable, familiar, and consistent.
- Try not to inadvertently reinforce or reward negative behavior. For example, if a pet learns that anxious pacing results in repeated invitations to snuggle on the forbidden couch, the pet may be more likely to continue the anxious behavior.
- Provide pets with positive reinforcement, such as attention and affection, when they are behaving in desirable ways. If Mr. Taylor allows Nellie to dictate the conditions of when and how she will eat, he will only reinforce the undesired behavior. Instead, he could offer Nellie a special treat or food when she eats where and when he wants her to. You want to catch the pet doing something right and then reinforce that desired behavior.
- Watch for changes in the dominance hierarchy when there are two or more surviving pets. This is particularly true if the pet who died was the dominant animal because the remaining animals often begin to compete for the dominant spot in the pecking order. The competition may involve growling, hissing, and even fighting, but the attacks usually do not result in injury. For the most part, help your clients understand that they should not punish their animals, but let them end the skirmishes on their own.
- Refrain from adopting a new animal "friend" for the surviving pet. This strategy usually backfires and there is no guarantee that any two animals will form a close, friendly relationship.

STEP 3 Stay Connected through Follow-up Care

- If the problems are serious or persist, refer clients to a veterinary or certified animal behaviorist or to a qualified animal trainer.
- Suggest that your client bring the surviving pet into your clinic for a physical examination to rule out any medical conditions that may be causing the behavior.

ROLE-PLAY IDEAS

For hospital managers and client care specialists: Practice talking with Mr. Taylor about his concerns for Nellie over Mack's death. Offer support and normalize his emotions.

For veterinary technicians: Act out a situation in which Mr. Taylor asks you point blank, "Do you think Nellie is grieving over Mack?" Practice what you would say and how you would approach the conversation.

For veterinarians: Respond to Mr. Taylor's concerns about Nellie and how he thinks Mack's death has affected her. Practice what you would say if Mr. Taylor asked: "Do you think Nellie is grieving for Mack? If so, what can I do to help her?" Provide support and follow-up.

Your Notes

SITUATION 14

Adopting New Pets

Mrs. Swenson and her family recently euthanized their beloved cat, Bruno. The entire family has been grieving, but now the children are starting to ask about the possibility of adopting a new cat. Mrs. Swenson tells you about the situation. She is unsure if she is ready for a new cat. She asks for your opinion about what she should do and what she should tell her children.

Assessment: What's Going On Here?

After a companion animal dies, many clients need time before they are ready to adopt a new pet. They may feel confused, guilty, and even angry when other people suggest it. It is not unusual for them to come to you for support. When a family instead of a single person is involved, as with the Swensons, the situation is complicated by the fact that different people are ready to take this step at different times. The grieving process is a very personal matter, and people in the same family may feel ready for a new companion animal at different times.

Plan

Support Protocol: What to Do, What to Say

STEP 1 Lay the Foundation

- Pet owners usually experience one of four basic reactions to the idea of adopting a new companion animal:
    1. They vow never to adopt a pet again.
    2. They vow to adopt a new pet as soon as possible.

3. They resign themselves to a period of grieving before they adopt a new pet, and then feel guilty when they finally bond again with a new companion animal.
4. They allow themselves the time they need to truly grieve, and then adopt a new pet when they feel ready to begin again.

- When a client's pet has died, try to determine which category the client falls into so you can provide appropriate support.

STEP 2 Implement Support Techniques

- The issue of adopting another pet often comes up in the follow-up calls made by a veterinary team member after a pet's death. Use the various communication skills you have learned (for example, active listening and paraphrasing) to help your client consider this option. Active listening is important because you may be able to discern whether the client is truly ready for a new pet.
- Educate the client about the reasons people usually have for wanting to adopt or not adopt a new pet following the death of another.
- Use your experience and skills to help clients think through the consequences of a decision they may make in haste.
- When the client is ready to adopt a new pet, assist him or her with the decision if you have the opportunity to do so. For example, you could suggest certain breeds that may be compatible with the client's lifestyle, answer questions about breeds, or provide printed materials or videos to view.
- For more examples of how to help a client think through this important decision, see the textbox "Providing Support for Clients on Pet Adoption."

STEP 3 Stay Connected through Follow-up Care

- It is not uncommon for pet owners to feel guilty once they have adopted a new pet and realize that they love it as much as they loved the one that died. Intense feelings for a new pet often make clients feel they are being disloyal to the pet that has died. You can help clients sort through their loyalty conflicts by letting them know that love is unlimited. Human beings are capable of loving more than one being at the same time, both living and dead. Clients also need to understand that they do not have to make a choice between loving the new pet and loving the pet that died. Instead, they can choose to love them both, in slightly different ways, just as parents can love more than one child.

- If a client is feeling guilty and disloyal about bonding with a new pet, you might also suggest "introducing" the new pet to the one that died by showing the new pet a photo of the former one, and talking out loud to the new pet about the former pet's habits and personality. This suggestion might sound silly, but pet owners who follow through usually feel relieved that they don't have to "choose" one pet over the other. They realize that they can continue to love the pet that died while bonding with the new pet in their lives.

Providing Support for Clients on Pet Adoption

Sometimes you must "listen between the lines" to your clients when they discuss adopting a new pet after a beloved pet has died. You can discern much about how clients' grief is progressing by what they say about this subject. You can help clients make this decision when it is the right time (and keep them from rushing into acquiring a new pet when they are not yet emotionally ready to take this step).

Pet owners who immediately adopt new pets are usually trying to avoid the sadness and loneliness of grief. You may hear a client say something like "I'm going out today to get a huge, gray tomcat who looks just like Jitters and I'm going to name him Jitters Jr." Comments like that should alert you to the possibility that clients may be trying to bring their pet back in the form of an identical new companion animal.

At the other end of the spectrum are clients who make comments like "I'll never get another cat. It's just too hard on me to lose them. Besides, I could never love another animal as much as I loved Jitters." Your first reaction to a comment like this is probably to say something like "Oh, you don't mean that! Think of all the animals out there who need good homes. The best thing for you right now would be to go out and adopt a new kitten."

However, this advice is almost never helpful. The "replacement philosophy" that commonly surrounds the death of a pet implies that companion-animal death is a relatively insignificant loss and that pets are easily replaced. In addition, giving advice, as opposed to active listening, tends to discount clients' feelings and stop further conversation.

continues

Providing Support for Clients on Pet Adoption, continued

When clients say they'll never own another pet, most don't really mean it. Rather, the comment reflects the grief they feel about this pet's death. If you acknowledge and validate your clients' feelings instead of trying to persuade them to feel otherwise, you'll provide more effective support. It's usually more effective to simply paraphrase your clients' comments, saying something like "It sounds like this loss is especially sad for you," or "I can hear that the thought of a new pet is not very comforting right now."

To help clients think through the consequences of a decision to adopt a new pet you might mention that, even though two pets may be of the same gender and breed, they will not necessarily have the same temperament. If the one that died was older, it may have been very mellow in temperament, whereas the new pet, if younger, may be more active. The new pet may also be untrained. The client may have thought of the pet that died as a confidant and protector, but the new pet may seem more like an unruly, needy child. In other words, the new pet can never really replace the old one; the client must be open to getting to know a new animal. When the client expects one thing from a companion animal but gets another, he or she may not be able to form an adequate bond with the new animal. Then, on top of the grief the client is already experiencing, he or she will feel a sense of guilt, especially if the client decides that he or she cannot provide the new pet with a loving home after all.

When grief progresses normally, a client begins to talk about getting a new pet in a positive way. The client will make a comment like "I miss having a dog in my house," or "I've always been intrigued with schnauzers. I might try that breed this time." Comments like these imply an interest in, rather than a desperate need for, a new pet. They tell you that the client has reached a stronger, more confident place in the grieving process and is now truly ready to explore the possibility of adopting a new pet.

ROLE-PLAY IDEAS

For hospital managers and client care specialists: Practice talking with Mrs. Swenson about her concerns over adopting a new pet. Normalize her emotions and answer her question about what you would do. Recruit other staff to practice dealing with an entire family who cannot all agree on the right time to adopt a new pet. Practice normalizing their emotions for themselves and for others.

For veterinary technicians: Normalize Mrs. Swenson's feelings and talk with her about the reasons many people have for adopting new pets. Carefully try to find out what the motivation is for different members of her family.

For veterinarians: Educate Mrs. Swenson about the motivations people have for wanting to adopt a new companion animal. Let her know that it's perfectly normal for family members not to agree about this at the same time. Gently help her explore what she thinks is motivating her children to want a new cat, and offer her support and follow-up assistance, including what to say to her children.

Your Notes

APPENIDIX

Forms

Grief Support Protocol

Purpose: ____

STEP 1 Lay the Foundation

_____ Prepare the physical environment.
_____ Stock client-education/support supplies.
_____ Assign/assume team member roles and responsibilities.

STEP 2 Implement Support Techniques

_____ Establish trust and rapport.
_____ Use a variety of appropriate verbal and nonverbal clinical communication skills and emotional support techniques.
_____ Provide clients with educational/support products, information, and referrals to take home.

STEP 3 Stay Connected through Follow-up Care

_____ Call clients within 24 hours to check on their well-being and clear up any questions or misunderstandings they might have.
_____ Send a handwritten condolence card or note as soon as possible.
_____ Schedule an appointment time if clients are picking up cremains and/or memorial pawprints. Ask if clients have questions or concerns they want to discuss.
_____ If case was unusual or especially emotional, debrief with team members, role-play, and review case at weekly staff meeting to improve everyone's client-support knowledge and skills and personal ability to draw closure to patient loss.

Role-Play Feedback Form

Name: ______________________________ Date: ____________________

Role-play situation:

____

____

____

____

____

Things that went well in the role-play:
(*to be filled out by colleagues observing the role-play*)

____

____

____

____

____

Ideas for improvement:
(*to be filled out by colleagues observing the role-play*)

____

____

____

____

____

Thank you for being willing to participate in this role-play. Your effort has helped all of us to learn! Great work!

Signed,

____

End-of-Life Referral Network

Resource	Contact Person	Contact Info
Local pet-loss counselor		
Local pet-loss support group		
Web/phone counselors		
Websites—before loss		
Websites—after loss		
Veterinary hospice program		
Home euthanasia practitioner		
Pet funeral home/cemetery		
Pet crematory		
Clergy		
Crisis hotline		
Suicide prevention		
Certified applied or veterinary animal behaviorist		
Trainer		
Animal control		
Local police/emergency		

Know your local resources, those on the Internet too! Update your list often and make multiple copies for your staff. Post a copy of your resource list by each computer and telephone and in every exam room so staff members have easy access to one when needed. It is also a good idea, as well as an appreciated service, to obtain business cards from your resource and referral network contacts and make them available to clients.

Resources

Professional Veterinary Organizations That Address Pet Loss Issues

American Animal Hospital Association (AAHA)

www.aahanet.org

Training materials for veterinary professionals; books/pamphlets for veterinary clients.

American Association for Human-Animal Bond Veterinarians (AAH-ABV)

http://aah-abv.org/net/home

Education, research, and support to enhance veterinarians' ability to create positive and ethical relationships among people, animals, and their environments.

American Veterinary Medicine Association (AVMA)

www.avma.org

Written guidelines for pet loss support services and veterinary hospice programs; brochures about pet and equine euthanasia.

Association for Veterinary Family Practice (AVFP)

www.avfp.org

Online and on-site (University of California–Davis) coursework in the emerging specialty of veterinary family practice. Topics include pets in families and society and the clinical skills needed to care for both patients and clients.

Delta Society

www.deltasociety.org

Improves human health through service and therapy animals.

International Association for Animal Hospice and Palliative Care (IAAHPC)

www.iaahpc.org

Interdisciplinary organization dedicated to promoting comfort-oriented nursing and medical care for companion animals as they near the end of their lives and as they die.

International Conference on Communication in Veterinary Medicine (ICCVM)

www.iccvm.com

Conference promoting the development of veterinary communication research and education. Often covers end-of-life communication.

International Society for Anthrozoology (ISAZ)

www.isaz.net

Scientific and scholarly study of human-animal interactions; *Anthrozoös* journal and professional meetings and conferences worldwide.

Pet Loss/Client Support Training Programs

Argus Institute

Colorado State University
James L. Voss Veterinary Teaching Hospital
300 West Drake
Fort Collins, CO 80525
Ph: 970-297-4143
argus@colostate.edu; www.argusinstitute.colostate.edu

Veterinary communication and grief support curriculum and training; Frank™ Workshop: workshop on veterinarian-client communication with continuing education credits available.

Association for Death Education and Counseling (ADEC)

111 Dear Lake Road, Suite 100
Deerfield, IL 60015
Ph: 847-509-0403
www.adec.org

National membership association providing certification and distance learning programs, as well as resources, information, and an annual conference.

Association for Pet Loss and Bereavement (APLB)

www.aplb.org

National organization providing training and "certification" for pet loss support counselors. The association's website offers information, counselor referrals, and online forums and support for pet owners.

Canadian Centre for Pet Loss Bereavement

www.petlosssupport.ca

Free public service website offering support, information, and training in pet loss counseling.

Center for Loss and Life Transition

www.centerforloss.com

Hosted by bereavement expert Dr. Alan Wolfelt with facilitation by Coleen Ellis, the center offers a "Pet Loss Companioning" Certification Program, as well as books and information about pet loss.

Institute for Healthcare Communication

555 Long Wharf Drive, 13th Floor

New Haven, CT 06511-5901

Ph: 800-800-5907, 203-772-8280

info@healthcarecomm.org; www.healthcarecomm.org

Nationally accredited, not-for-profit organization that trains physicians and, in recent years, veterinarians throughout North America in effective communication skills, euthanasia procedures, and the like.

Helpful Books on Providing Pet Loss Support

Barton Ross, C., and J. Baron-Sorenson. *Pet Loss and Human Emotion: A Guide to Recovery*, 2nd ed. New York: Routledge, 2007.

Carmack, B. J. *Grieving the Death of a Pet*. Minneapolis: Augsburg Fortress, 2003.

Cornell, K., J. Brandt, and K. A. Bonvicini, guest eds. "Effective Communication in Veterinary Practice." Pp. xv–xvi in *Veterinary Clinics of North America: Small Animal Practice*, vol. 37, no. 1. Philadelphia: W. B. Saunders, 2007.

Durrance, D., and L. Lagoni. *Connecting with Clients: Practical Communication for 10 Common Situations*, 2nd ed. Lakewood, CO: AAHA Press, 2010.

Lagoni, L., C. Butler, and S. Hetts. *The Human-Animal Bond and Grief*. Philadelphia: W. B. Saunders, 1994.

Odendaal, Johannes. *Pets and Our Mental Health: The Why, the What, and the How*. New York: Vantage Press, 2002.

Stern, M., and S. Cropper. *Loving and Losing a Pet: A Psychologist and a Veterinarian Share Their Wisdom*. Lanham, MD: Rowman and Littlefield, 1998.

Helpful Books about Pet Loss for Children

Morehead, D. *A Special Place for Charlee*. Broomfield, CO: Partners in Publishing, 1996.

Rylant, C. *Cat Heaven*. New York: Blue Sky Press, 1997.

———. *Dog Heaven*. New York: Blue Sky Press, 1995.

Veterinary Grief Counselors

Deborah Antinori, MA, LPC, CT

Author of *Journey through Pet Loss*, audiobook

Ph: 908-766-0110

dantinori@gmail.com; www.petlossaudio.com

Argus Institute

Colorado State University

James L. Voss Veterinary Teaching Hospital

300 West Drake

Fort Collins, CO 80525

Ph: 970-297-4143

argus@colostate.edu; www.argusinstitute.colostate.edu/whatnow.htm

Clinical service providing client grief support

Dana Durrance, MA

Veterinary Grief Specialist and Consultant

dldurrance@msn.com

Dana is a veterinary grief specialist and offers support and consultations for veterinary professionals who need help and support in working with grieving clients.

Stephanie LaFarge, PhD

Senior Director of Counseling Services

ASPCA Counseling Services

1717 South Philo Road, Suite 36

Urbana, IL 61802

Ph: 217-337-9773; cell: 877-GRIEF-10 (877-474-3310)

stephaniel@aspca.org

The ASPCA Pet Loss Hotline (PLH) is available 24/7, nationwide. There is no charge for the service, and no information that could identify the caller is required, just the first name of the caller and the name of the pet.

Marty Touseley

Certified Hospice Bereavement Counselor

www.griefhealing.com

Supportive information and "A Different Grief: Coping with Pet Loss," a 24-lesson e-course for pet parents who've lost a pet. Supplemental material for supporting grieving children is also available.

World by the Tail, Inc.

126 West Harvard Street, Suite 5

Fort Collins, CO 80525, Ph: 888-271-8444

info@wbtt.com; www.veterinarywisdomforpetparents.com

How-to information about end-of-life planning and preparation as it relates to pet loss. Up-to-date referrals, resources, consultation, and products for pet parents and mental health professionals who provide pet loss support; VeterinaryWisdom™ Support Center; free e-books and client handouts about pet loss.

University Helplines

Please see current listings in each issue of the *Journal of the American Veterinary Association*, or visit www.veterinarywisdomforpetparents.com for up-to-date contact information.

Providers of Memorials and Client Support Products

Argus Institute

Colorado State University

James L. Voss Veterinary Teaching Hospital

300 West Drake, Fort Collins, CO 80525

Ph: 970-297-4143

argus@colostate.edu; www.argusinstitute.colostate.edu/whatnow.htm

What Now booklet for grieving pet owners; clinical service providing client grief support; Veterinary Pet Hospice Program.

Center for Loss and Life Transition

www.centerforloss.com

When Your Pet Dies: A Guide to Mourning, Remembering, and Healing, by bereavement expert Dr. Alan Wolfelt.

In-Home Pet Euthanasia Directory

www.inhomepeteuthanasia.com

State-by-state directory of veterinarians offering in-home euthanasia services. Listings are managed by Dr. Kathleen Cooney of Home to Heaven, P.C., a mobile pet euthanasia service in northern Colorado.

Pawz2Remember

James Willett

321 West Belden Avenue, #1E

Chicago, IL 60614-3851

www.pawz2remember.com

Keepsake jewelry made from pets' collars and tags; service may be offered through veterinary practices.

Pet Angel World Services

2040 Boston Road, Suite 20

Wilbraham, MA 01095

Ph: 413-543-1144

www.PetAngelWorldServices.com

Up-to-date information about the pet cremation industry and how it impacts pet owners and veterinarians; grief support resources; pet funeral and memorial services; resources for veterinarians.

World by the Tail, Inc.

126 West Harvard Street, Suite 5

Fort Collins, CO 80525

Ph: 888-271-8444

info@wbtt.com; www.veterinarywisdom.com

ClayPaws™ pawprint kits and other pet tribute products; condolence cards, grief education card enclosures, and We Care brochures; Body Care Bags—polyethylene ziplock bags with "A Pet's Love Is Forever" imprint; VeterinaryWisdom™ Resource Center; up-to-date referrals, resources, consultation, and products for pet parents and veterinary professionals who provide pet loss support.

Glossary

acknowledge: to recognize the existence or truth of something.

active listening: to listen for feelings rather than for the factual content of conversations.

anticipatory grief: the grief that occurs prior to an actual loss or death. Examples of pet loss situations that may trigger anticipatory grief include aging pets and pets who are terminally ill. The symptoms of anticipatory grief include any or all of the symptoms of normal grief.

attending: body language that lets the person who is talking know that careful attention is being paid to what is being said.

body language: the gestures, movements, and mannerisms by which a person or animal communicates with others.

clinical communication skills: specific verbal and nonverbal techniques and methods used to convey knowledge or emotional support in a clinical setting.

comfort: to strengthen; a physical, mental, and/or emotional state of ease of well-being.

communicate: to convey knowledge of or information about; to make known.

complicated grief: grief that is more difficult than usual as a result of the circumstances surrounding a death. Examples of factors that often complicate grief for pet owners are feelings of responsibility for a pet's accidental death, feelings of guilt after deciding to euthanize a pet, and the general tendency for society to trivialize companion animal death.

confidentiality: an ethical commitment to keep shared information private.

demonstration: the visual display, act, or process of showing, usually accompanied by verbal explanation.

empathy: an intellectual and emotional comprehension of another person's condition without actually experiencing the other person's feelings.

euthanasia, client-present: a medical procedure during which pet owners witness the humane termination of an animal's life. During the procedure, pet owners' needs and grief responses are attended to in a sensitive and compassionate manner. The use of ritual, ceremony, and effective helping strategies is encouraged in order to promote positive grief outcomes for survivors.

gentle confrontation: method of pointing out the discrepancies or inconsistencies in what someone has said or done. Gentle confrontation may take the form of a question or a statement.

giving permission: encouraging clients to think, feel, and behave however they need to—for example, in response to grief, which is unique to each person—within safe limits, without fear of judgment.

grief: the normal way to adjust to endings and changes, such as the death of a loved one. Grief is a necessary process for healing emotional wounds.

helping: providing short-term assistance, mainly in the form of information and comfort, to others at a time when they are in need of such assistance, such as before, during, and after the death of a loved one.

human-animal bond: a popular way of referring to the types of relationships and attachments people form with animals, particularly companion animals. Also, an accepted area of scholarly research.

immediacy: the combination of gentle confrontation and self-disclosure to comment on unspoken feelings or thoughts that currently exist within an interpersonal relationship.

loss: an ending or a point of change or transition. Loss can be permanent, as in death, or temporary, as in the loss of a job.

mourning: a synonym for grief often applying to the outward expressions and behaviors displayed following a loss and the period of time during which it is more socially acceptable to show the outward signs of grief.

nonverbal communication: communication that is conveyed without words through facial expressions, body postures, gestures, and hand movements, as well as through writing, reading, and listening.

normalizing: lending credibility to others' thoughts, feelings, behaviors, and experiences. Often this takes the form of verbal communication that reassures another person that his or her behavior fits the situation and is to be expected.

paraphrase: the restatement or summary of another person's communication in order to test the receiver's understanding of these comments.

primary loss: the actual loss of something or someone and the main cause of grief. An example in terms of pet loss is the actual death of a companion animal.

questions: inquiries that elicit more detailed information and create opportunities for others to talk in more depth about what they are experiencing. *Open-ended* questions begin with "how" or "what" rather than with "why." *Closed-ended* questions can be responded to with "yes," "no," "fine," or some other one- or two-word answer.

rapport: relationship marked by trust and harmony.

secondary losses: disruptions and changes in a person's life that are due to a primary loss. An example in terms of pet loss is the loss of routine and shared activity, such as walks or participation in competitive shows, that occurs when a companion animal dies.

self-disclosure: the brief sharing of a similar or related personal experience through a verbal or written account when it may be appropriate and of use to the listener or reader.

structuring the environment: adapting the physical elements of an environment to better meet the situation at hand.

support: in the context of the grieving process, a method of actively listening to another's nonmedical concerns without taking action to solve the problem.

support protocol: an agreed-upon or known plan that allows people, such as veterinary team members, to work together to provide emotional support for clients experiencing grief or other pet-related challenges.

surrogate grief: grief that belongs to one person (e.g., a pet owner), but is experienced or carried by someone else (e.g., a shelter worker or a veterinary professional), as a result of the owner's absence, indifference, or inability to grieve.

symbolic loss: a loss that is associated with a previous loss in life. An example in terms of pet loss is the loss of a pet associated with a special person, place, thing, or time in life (e.g., a spouse who has died, or a marriage that has ended). The pet's death ends the link. Although pet loss is significant in its own right, the grief owners feel because of a symbolic loss is often more intense.

touch: in the context of the grieving process, comfort, care, and concern demonstrated by the use of physical contact.

trust: faith, confidence, and reliance on the ability, strength, character, or truth of someone or something.

unresolved grief: grief that occurs when free expression of normal grief is prevented or when, for some reason, the normal grief process is arrested or blocked. Unresolved or unfinished issues due to an earlier, significant loss are frequently restimulated during pet loss, causing many pet owners to struggle with the impact of a past loss during their pet loss experiences.

verbal communication: communication skills and techniques that make use of the spoken word.

About the Authors

LAUREL LAGONI is president and CEO of World by the Tail, Inc.; the creator and distributor of ClayPaws™, the original pawprint kit; and the director of the Veterinary Wisdom™ Support Center at www.veterinarywisdomforpet parents.com. Previously, Laurel was the cofounder and director of the Argus Institute for Families and Veterinary Medicine at Colorado State University's James L. Voss Veterinary Teaching Hospital. Laurel holds a bachelor's degree in journalism from Iowa State University and a master's degree in human development and family studies, with specialties in family therapy and grief education, from Colorado State University.

Laurel is the coauthor of four books, including the groundbreaking text *The Human-Animal Bond and Grief* (W.B. Saunders, 1994). She has written more than fifty book chapters and journal articles and has been an invited speaker at numerous national veterinary conferences. She has also lectured at the Smithsonian Institute in Washington, D.C. Laurel contributed to *Chicken Soup for the Pet Lover's Soul* and has been showcased on ABC's *20/20* program. Fort Collins, Colorado, is Laurel's home, where she lives with her husband, two daughters, and several dogs and cats.

DANA DURRANCE is a veterinary grief specialist and consultant. She holds two bachelor's degrees from the University of Colorado (one in communication, and the other in psychology). She also holds a master's degree in clinical psychology from the University of Colorado and is the former director of the nationally renowned "Changes: Support for People and Pets" program at Colorado State University's James L. Voss Veterinary Teaching Hospital.

For the past fifteen years, Dana has lectured at veterinary conferences, veterinary hospitals, schools, and individual veterinary practices all over the country (and in Europe). As well as writing books, she publishes regularly in veterinary journals. She has a monthly column on the veterinary practice website ImproMed.com and is the grief specialist for PetAngelWorldService .com. She is a regular speaker at Alameda East Veterinary Hospital (home of Animal Planet's *Emergency Vets*) and has also appeared as a grief specialist on ABC's *Good Morning America*.

Dana lives in Colorado Springs, Colorado, with her husband (a veterinarian) and together they own Mountain Shadows Pet Hospital, an AAHA-accredited veterinary hospital. They have a daughter, a son, and two dogs. As both a pet loss counselor and a veterinary practice owner, she has special insight into both pet owners and veterinary professionals.